Reflective Practice

Key Themes in Health and Social Care series

Nick J. Fox, The Body

Reflective Practice

Janet Hargreaves and Louise Page

polity

First published in 2013 by Polity Press

Polity Press
65 Bridge Street
Cambridge CB2 1UR, UK

Polity Press
350 Main Street
Malden, MA 02148, USA

ISBN-13: 978-0-7456-5423-2
ISBN-13: 978-0-7456-5424-9 (pb)

A catalogue record for this book is available from the British Library.

Typeset in 10.25 on 13pt Scala by
Servis Filmsetting Ltd, Stockport, Cheshire

For further information on Polity, visit our website: www.politybooks.com

Contents

Figures

Tables

Boxes

Acknowledgements

Writing this book together has been a great journey, uniting our different experiences and ideas. It has been helped by encouragement and critique from family and friends, in particular Richard Hargreaves, who has patiently drafted and re-drafted the original diagrams and made, photographed and helped to eat the Knickerbocker Glory.

Introduction

This book is written for students and qualified professionals who want to extend their knowledge, skills and understanding of reflective practice. This book does not seek to focus on any one discipline, because reflection is shared by all professional groups. It is written by Janet, an academic with nursing qualifications, and Louise, a professional writer with academic support experience. We both use reflection in our teaching and everyday life. We are sure that reflective practice can have a positive and confidence-boosting role in all aspects of professional learning and will illustrate this through the stories in the book.

Looking at the literature, every health and social care discipline has a motivation for using reflection. Development of life-long learning is highlighted for medical students (Barley, 2012) as the vast knowledge base required for practice cannot all be learned and remembered, but this sentiment is true of all professions as research and legislation leads to rapid change: all of us need the ability to find things out for ourselves and learn from our experience. Understanding how to learn is explored in most detail in the literature from teacher education, and so we draw on this regularly throughout the book. The development of empathy and self-awareness also features in many justifications for the teaching of reflective practice, for example in health care (Bulman & Schutz, 2008), social work (Brookfield, 2009) medicine and dentistry (Brett-MacLean, Cave, Yiu, Kelner & Ross, 2010; Brown, 2010).

In different ways, the literature suggests that reflection and reflective practice help professionals to develop and critique their own practice. By deliberately choosing literature that comes from as many professional viewpoints from health and social care as we could find, as well as teacher education, we hope to show the universality of the concepts involved. What became clear to us was that each profession values reflection and reflective practice in different ways. For many of the texts written about medicine and dentistry, reflection was promoted as a necessary tool for helping with complex decision making and with the tension between the clinical and the personal. For teachers it seems to be more cerebral; a process that helps teachers to learn to learn, and thus to help others. For health and social work, intuitive and self-reflective behaviour is already assumed so there is more focus on deeper personal reflection and critical reflection, looking at the socio-political aspects of practice. This difference seemed helpful and enlightening to us, reflecting perhaps the discourses identified by Mantzoukas & Watkinson who say: 'In the process of learning a discipline, individuals have to be able to differentiate themselves from others while remaining part of a social context' (Mantzoukas & Watkinson, 2008, p. 130).

Using a series of examples and templates, we will guide you through reflective practice in a variety of situations. Our emphasis is on practicalities. We recognize that the majority of people in health and social care disciplines are 'hands on' and kinaesthetic learners. Sharing stories is a powerful tool for learning. Using stories and drawing on academic literature, we have collected ideas, exercises and theoretical situations to develop skills for the learning, understanding and recording of reflective practice. We feel that reflective practice is strongly linked to ethics and professional judgement, so these feature throughout the book, not as add-ons, but embedded in everyday reflection.

In chapters 1, 2 and 3, we introduce you to reflection and reflective practice, including background, models and a timeline for development.

Chapters 4, 5 and 6 look at three different 'how to' aspects:

writing reflection, particularly where you might need to write for an academic assessment; reflecting in groups; and reflecting in other ways, such as through walking, and using the environment around you.

Chapters 7 and 8 take reflection in different directions. Chapter 7 looks at situations where an individual professional may be in trouble, and the ways in which reflection can help to avoid, and recover from, personal difficulties. Chapter 8 looks at the awkward, dangerous questions that reflection can lead to, and how you might manage these in practice.

Chapter 9 offers some of the cases against and barriers to reflection: the arguments that it is 'just thinking', makes no difference to practice and cannot be assessed are reviewed and suggestions made.

Finally, we conclude by bringing together the themes of the book and our personal reflection on writing it.

CHAPTER ONE

Reflection in context: what this book is all about

Chapter Summary

Reflection is promoted for effective development in every professional code and educational course that you will come across in your career. This chapter will set the scene for the book; locating reflective practice within the recent historical development of professional education. Through studying this chapter and engaging in the exercises, you will be able to:

- discuss the place of reflective practice in professional education
- identify the significance of storytelling to understanding practice
- make connections between your personal beliefs, your practice and major ethical theories
- reflect on the application of reflective skills to your own professional practice and development.

Introduction

What does it mean to reflect, or to be a 'reflective practitioner'? Is it innate, a personal way of being or learning style? Alternatively, is it something you can learn, develop and improve?

In this book, we are going to help you to discover what reflective practice is, to develop your reflective abilities, to express your reflection in ways that other people can understand

1

and to successfully demonstrate your reflection when used for assessment. Throughout this book, we do not have any particular profession in mind. Louise is not qualified in any health or social care profession; she has worked with and supported health and social care students, and writes plays about health and illness. Janet is a nurse by background; she works in higher education in a multi-professional setting. We draw on literature from health, medicine, social work, dentistry and education, in fact from any discipline that we think adds to understanding and offers useful ideas. Naturally, we draw on our own experience but we use stories and illustrations from many professional viewpoints, in order to demonstrate that reflection crosses inter-professional language and practice.

In order to start on this journey, we want to offer three areas for consideration:

(1) A short history of reflective practice, where it came from and why it has become so important.
(2) The use of stories – storytelling is a powerful medium for reflection. It offers a structure in which to narrate actual events, but also the freedom to explore safely thoughts and feelings that may be taboo. We will frequently use stories in this book and will help you to develop your own skills of narration.
(3) Ethical practice – questions about what is the right way to behave are rarely far from view when we engage in reflection. There is no single way to decide on the most ethical course of action and frequently no perfect answers. Here we will explain ethical theories and suggest one framework we think is particularly suitable for thinking about ethics as you reflect on your practice.

A short history of reflective practice

The industrial revolution is probably as good a starting place for this as any. In the nineteenth century, the mechanization of just about everything from transport to food production changed the way people all over the world worked and lived their lives. Central to this revolution was the application of scientific methods – if you can observe and measure, then you can predict and control. The effects of this scientific explosion were not just concerned with factories or industry; the philosophy behind them infiltrated every aspect of human life. In medicine, health and social care, the human condition was investigated, dissected, measured and categorized.

A great deal of good has come from these developments. In medicine, the discovery of bacteria and viruses has transformed our understanding of disease (Le Fanu, 1999). Psychological research has led to greater understanding of how the human mind works, revolutionizing the care of people who are mentally ill (Rodham, 2010), and theories from sociology have given us ways of explaining and predicting human behaviour (Cohen & Kennedy, 2007).

However, the downside to this focus on science was that, by the twentieth century, its dominance was such that knowledge gained from scientific methods seemed more important than any other sort of knowledge. Many people challenged this view, but it was Donald Schön's seminal work, published originally in 1983 and 1987, that challenged the scientific method in professional education (Schön, 1991): reflective practice was born.

Schön's argument goes like this:

The cliff top and the swamp

Imagine you are with a group of people who are on a journey (see figure 1.1). You come to a cliff top and can see a range of possible destinations in the distance. You need to decide on the correct destination and best route to get there. The various paths below you are clear to see; you can trace each one, plan ahead, decide on a direction and continue on your way.

Another group of people are also trying to reach their destination, but they are starting from the bottom of the cliff,

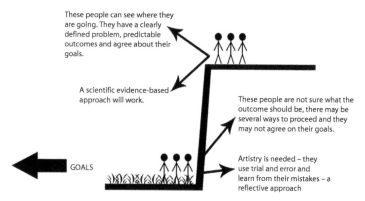

These people can see where they are going. They have a clearly defined problem, predictable outcomes and agree about their goals.

A scientific evidence-based approach will work.

These people are not sure what the outcome should be, there may be several ways to proceed and they may not agree on their goals.

GOALS

Artistry is needed – they use trial and error and learn from their mistakes – a reflective approach

Figure 1.1 The cliff top and the swamp (adapted from Schön, 1991)

where the ground is swampy. They cannot see clearly ahead and the destination is out of sight, so they do not know which may be the best path to take. They use trial and error, learning from their mistakes and picking up new information as they pick their way carefully through the swamp.

For Schön, the scientific approach available to the cliff-top people, which he calls 'technical rationality', is fine where problems have definition and clarity, outcomes are predictable and all the people involved have shared goals. However, he claims that problems in professional life are rarely this simple. We are often uncertain about what the problems might be, have limited research to guide us, and disagree about what the best course of action is. In these situations, the skills developed by the swamp people are much more effective. This – the 'artistry' of professional practice – is the skill-set Schön sought to teach, develop and constantly improve through reflective practice.

A reversal of priorities

Schön looked around him and started to analyse the way in which professionals were educated. He noticed a hierarchy in highly regarded professions where the most attention and value were given to theory, followed by application of knowledge, and finally by skills and everyday practice. For example, a barrister or attorney studied the theory of law for several years before having the opportunity to practise, and medical students studied anatomy and physiology long before they met their first patient. As professions with an apprentice basis, such as allied health and social work, nursing and midwifery, aspired to greater professional status, they too began to adopt these principles. Much has changed in professional education in the last few decades, the privileging of theoretical learning over practice learning is no longer as common and most professional courses include at least some development of the skills and artistry of the profession right from the start. It may therefore seem that the trend has been reversed.

Or has it?

Despite these changes, professions remain very guarded and defend the 'knowledge' that they see as central to their unique practice. Think about the last place you worked, or attended for a placement. Who earned the most money, had the most power or gained the most respect as a professional person? It is much more likely that this person also had the longest period of education and the most academic qualifications.

Evidence-based or research-based practice still privileges quantitative rather than qualitative methods of enquiry. Projects that use scientific methods, for example predicting the probability of a cause-and-effect relationship, or the effectiveness of a new policy, treatment or drug, are more likely to gain funding.

So, whilst there has been a great deal of change, there remains ambivalence about the place of the artistry or craft basis of professional behaviour.

Deconstructing reflective practice

Schön went on to try to identify the successful activities undertaken by the swamp people that helped them to think well professionally. It is probably easiest to illustrate these using two examples.

Example 1: a child learning a skill

Activity	Analysis
A sunny day in the park; a young child is poised at the top of a sloping grassy bank about to cycle down it without trainer wheels for the first time. The adult observing from a distance sees much theory is evident. Forces of gravity, mass, kinetic energy and velocity act on the child and the bike's frame as s/he shakily proceeds down the hill. The focus is on staying upright but the presence of 'theory in use' is all around.	Theory in use
Despite being young, s/he already brings a wealth of knowledge to the problem. S/he knows how to coordinate limbs and eyes to progress forward, and to shift body weight from left to right to avoid falling. S/he has also already mastered the art of steering using the handlebars whilst riding with trainer wheels. The child will probably not be able to articulate an understanding of gravity but knowledge of its effect is evident from observed behaviour. This 'knowledge in use' is added to and refined every time s/he gets onto the bike.	Knowledge in use
The child is absolutely focused on the task in hand – in the moment, s/he concentrates, appraises how well s/he is doing, adjusts balance, speed and steering.	Reflection in action
Arriving shakily at the bottom of the hill, the child thinks back over the event – powerful feelings of pride at staying upright and relief at not being too badly hurt – a few cuts and grazes but nothing worse! S/he thinks about what was good and how to improve – the adults give praise, ask questions about feelings and give feedback on performance – this greatly enhances the child's ability to 'reflect on action'.	Reflection on action

Activity	Analysis
Many cycle rides later, we see this young person riding through town. Mastery of the bike is evident as we watch a skilfully, smoothly executed turn at speed: observing traffic, wind speed, road conditions, pot holes and pedestrians, our cyclist rides the bike with ease. This thoughtful, engaged, confident cycling is an example of 'reflective practice' – learning continues with every journey taken and the skill is evident in the performance.	Reflective practice!

The years roll on –

Example 2: the child is now the adult

Activity	Analysis
Our young person is now an adult, engaged in a professional conversation. Theories of communication are evident in body language, eye contact and verbal and non-verbal communication techniques.	Theory in use
The person in conversation is showing anger – raised voice, wide gestures, aggressive stance. Our professional sits back a little, uses open body language, active listening and questions to understand and dissipate the angry response – knowledge in action is evident from the behaviour displayed.	Knowledge in use
S/he may look relaxed but inside his/her mind is racing: 'How am I doing?' 'What should I say next?' 'What questions will get the best reaction?' 'What has worked before?' S/he engages in a constant internal narrative, appraising feelings and combining theoretical understanding and experience; reflecting in the moment helps to navigate through a potentially difficult situation.	Reflection in action
Reflecting back on the encounter, our professional analyses his/her skills and the outcomes of the conversation. S/he is excited and pleased to have managed a difficult situation well, but by narrating the event to a supervisor more can be learned. The supervisor asks probing questions offering challenges and alternative views.	Reflection on action

Activity	Analysis
This professional is a reflective practitioner – engaged, open to learning and self-aware, each professional encounter helping to learn and improve on performance.	Reflective practice!

 EXERCISE

Think back to the last time you were working in your professional role. It may have been the first time you had met a person and you were assessing their needs, or you were with a person you know well and have a regular professional appointment with, or maybe a teaching or management issue that you were dealing with. Jot down your thoughts on the questions below:

➢ Theory – what theoretical ideas underpin the episode you are thinking about?
➢ Knowledge – what knowledge was evident in your behaviour?
➢ Reflection in action – think back to what you did and said, how you felt, what was going through your mind at the time; how did you decide how to act in a particular way, what to say, or not to say?
➢ Reflection on action – looking back now, how do you feel about the episode? Did it go as well as it could have, what went well and why – can you use this learning again? What were you less pleased with, and what would you change if you could?
➢ Stop at this point and look again at what you have written. If you have the opportunity to do so, ask a friend or colleague if they will listen to your story and ask you questions about it. Does what you have written surprise you? Does the telling of the story, either to yourself by writing it down or verbally to another, reveal anything to you that you could not see before? Be honest – are there things you have omitted or embellished? Why?

Reflection and professional education

So far so good – but how often do you actually do this in your everyday practice? When practice becomes familiar, it is easy to drop into a routine where we no longer have this heightened awareness. Just like the cyclist earlier, we fall into automatic routines, so it may only be when something unexpected or worrying occurs that we are jolted back into thinking more critically. Supporters of reflective practice say that developing reflective skills can harness the learning in everyday practice as well as in critical moments, aiding personal development and improving skills.

 TIME FOR REFLECTION

Did you find this exercise easy or difficult? In chapter 2, we will introduce you to ways of structuring your reflection, using a number of models.

Schön, along with many other theorists, continued to develop their ideas, which have been progressively adopted and embedded into professional education and development through the late twentieth and early twenty-first centuries. People researching professional behaviour also began making theoretical links between being reflective and expert practice. The work of Patricia Benner (Benner, 1984; Benner, Chesla & Tanner, 2009) has been particularly influential, not just within nursing – the subject of her research – but across professional education generally. In her original (1984) research, Benner used Critical Incident Technique to gain insights into the everyday practice of nurses. From this, she developed a model of skill acquisition that uses the work of Dreyfus and Dreyfus, who contribute a chapter in her later work (Dreyfus & Dreyfus, 2009). This suggests that, through a combination of education and practice, practitioners progress from novice, where theoretical knowledge is used under supervision, to expert in five stages, which, like the swampy lowlands in Schön, require experience and artistry for success (see table 1.1).

Many texts make links between gaining such professional expertise and reflective practice. For example, McCracken and Marsh (2008) show the importance of critical reflective thought to applying expertise to evidence-based practice in social work, whilst Bulman and Schutz (2008) identify the development and importance of reflection in nursing. There are also an increasing

Table 1.1 Skill acquisition from novice to expert (Dreyfus & Dreyfus, 2009)	
Novice	The learner is inexperienced. At this stage the learner gains theoretical knowledge and learns rules – such as following instructions or a recipe for action. The cyclist in the example above demonstrates basic rules of handling the bike, and road safety. The professional would have learned about the rules of verbal and non-verbal communication.
Advanced beginner	The learner now practises these skills and begins to recognize patterns, and the various aspects of the skill. They may still fall back on 'how to' rules and make frequent mistakes, and can be frustrated by uncertainty and complexity. The cyclist may cope in a straight line but not round corners; the communicator may be gaining good speaking skills but be unable to watch for non-verbal cues at the same time.
Competent	This is the stage when the learner has embedded, or learned, the rules and begins to reach out. In real practice, simply following a set of rules is rarely sufficient. Soon you are in the position of having to decide which rule to follow first, or which is most appropriate. Usually you are dealing with more than one situation at a time, so, like the cyclist, just being able to ride the bike is not enough. The learner uses experience, trial and error, success and failure, leading to greater skill and understanding.
Proficient	With greater experience our learner is now more able to make decisions intuitively and perform with skill and ease. Seeing beyond the immediate issues, and being able to draw on wide practice and knowledge, the communicator will recognize distress or anger and start to use skills to address and manage this, before things get out of hand.
Expert	The expert knows what needs to be achieved, and how to do this in a range of complex and uncertain settings. They no longer ride a bike, they just ride – bike and human in harmony. Similarly, communication is no longer a set of learned rules, but is a complex embedded interaction. Experts can, of course, make mistakes, but they are generally able to perform smoothly and with confidence.

number of papers making links between reflection and decision making for medicine – see, for example, Balla, Heneghan, Glasziou, Thompson and Balla (2009) and Graber (2009). All suggest that using the seemingly 'soft' skills of reflection can enhance professional practice in many settings.

Although the basis of this assumption – that reflection is always a 'good thing' – can be challenged (see chapter 9), for now we will use this as the starting point for exploration. Our reason for this is that, in the wake of the assertion that it *is* a good thing, regulated medical, health and social care professions began to see reflection and reflective practice as a hallmark of good professional behaviour. They now require it to be embedded into education courses, requirements for continued registration / licence to practise, and Continuing Professional Development. Like it or not, reflective practice is here to stay.

Storytelling

Storytelling is something that all people do – we use stories to explain, construct and understand our lives. Even if you are very new to your chosen profession, you will already have found that there is a strong oral tradition in health and social care professions whereby colleagues often tell stories ('my worst day', 'my most embarrassing moment'). It is not surprising then that reflective practice often revolves around storytelling. In this book we have already used several stories – Schön uses 'the cliff top and the swamp' (see figure 1.1) to make sense of how professionals need to think if they are to be successful, and you have thought of stories from your own life or professional practice to do the exercises.

What is a story? Stephen King says that stories have a plot and are in three parts (King, 2001, p. 187):

Narration: 'this moves the story from a to b and so on to z'
Description: what happened when and how
Dialogue: the voices and words of the various characters.

These three devices draw the reader through the story. To illustrate this, here is a story from Janet's experience of learning to nurse:

Janet's First Nights

When she trained as a nurse in the 1970s in England you were apprenticed to a hospital, undertaking three-month periods of clinical work interspersed with month-long 'blocks' in nursing school. After eight weeks of basic theory, she went on her first ward, female surgical, and after about six weeks, did her first two-week period on night duty. They were taking emergencies one night and an elderly woman with acute abdominal pain was admitted. The doctor on duty asked for her to be starved, for an intravenous drip to be inserted, and for a naso-gastric tube to be passed, thus enabling her digestive system to be rested. Janet knew this procedure theoretically but had never actually seen one passed, let alone done one herself. The qualified nurse from an adjacent ward told her to set up her trolley, went through to check she had the right equipment and to observe that she safely passed the tube into her patient's stomach – not her lung! The nurse stood in silence at the end of the bed and watched Janet: either the poor patient was remarkably compliant or she really felt too ill to resist, so the tube went in with no difficulty and Janet spent a while sitting with her as several litres of fluid drained from her stressed digestive system.

As King says, this story has a 'plot' and a beginning, middle and end; it then narrates what happened and introduces the four characters. It conforms to many types of story that we have seen repeated often in professional practice in that it is both a 'my first placement' story and a 'rite of passage' story. It is also what Plummer describes as an 'epiphany' – that is, a story that conveys a moment of realization or change (Plummer, 2001).

It attempts to convey what was an authentic experience at that time, including some of the feelings Janet remembers experiencing regarding the relationship between student nurse, doctor, patient and qualified nurse. It also contains some, but not all, of the characteristics of Schön's reflective practice elements introduced earlier in this chapter in that *theory in use* and *knowledge in action* are evident. However, it gives the reader no insight into Janet's thoughts or reflections; this was not something she discussed or thought about at the time.

It is an honest and faithful account but it is not verifiable as 'true'. Knowing that stories are fiction helps to remind us that reflective accounts can never be exactly true of, or a perfect substitute for, the actual experience. Even factual accounts in newspapers and autobiographical writing are only proxy for the real thing and are subject to interpretation and challenge. We tell stories differently for different audiences. For example, you would relate your first date to a friend, a parent or your subsequent partner differently: the story may be the same, but the meaning you wish the listener to take from it will be different.

You may be wondering why storytelling matters. We believe that being aware that you are writing a story, and understanding how to do this well, will improve your ability to structure and share your reflections with others. In your reflective writing, you may be required to present something that is factual, such as that you were working on a certain day and that certain things happened, but the narration of this event will change depending on who you are telling it to, why, and how much time has elapsed since then.

The story of 'Janet's first nights' is told decades after the event, and has been re-told periodically since. The pattern of night duty, the geography of the ward and the sketch of the events is a faithful account, but much of the detail is lost to time, memory and the re-telling of the story. At the time, Janet may well have recounted this as a positive example of her coping skills – she had what it took to be a 'good' nurse – resourceful, competent and successful: *Look at me! I was left in charge on nights and passed my first naso-gastric tube!* Now she tells it to illustrate how much has changed, particularly when faced with nostalgia for a lost 'golden age' of health care: *Look at me! Left to manage a ward full of ill people with just a few months' training!* Finally, the story is re-told in this book.

You are not writing or reflecting to entertain or to make a living, but to convey your experience and the process of learning to yourself and third parties. Indeed, the very act of writing reflection may alter your perception (Bolton, 2010). You will not be judged on your creative abilities, but writing your story/narrative with some confidence and clarity will help you to present your work well and to express your ideas clearly. Just as the 'academic essay' is a written form that can be learned, and improved, writing reflectively can be learned and improved too. In chapter 2, we will help you to construct your own reflective stories, and in chapter 4 to write for reflection.

Ethics

The final area that we want to introduce as a core element of this book is ethical decision making for reflective practice. Health and social care practitioners are always working within an ethical context: whether it is the 'big' decisions, such as taking a child away from his/her parents or life-threatening treatment options, or the 'everyday' allocation of time and resources, there is always a decision to be made and dilemmas over the right course of action.

We believe that you cannot practise reflectively without considering these ethical elements: reflective practice *is* ethical practice. However, any ethical textbook or a cursory review of current affairs will show you that this is a complex area and that the range of approaches to ethical practice is confusing and contradictory. Here we want to offer you a brief overview of ethical theories and outline one of these approaches that we believe is particularly useful when exploring reflective practice.

Ethics is not something that you can learn easily from a book. Its origins lie in moral philosophy, in the debates that people have had over thousands of years about the right way for humans to live effectively together and to flourish. Ethics describes the theories, principles and rules that we create to try to order our societies, businesses and personal behaviour (Beauchamp & Childress, 2013). Your profession is bound by a code that draws on moral philosophy, outlining behaviour that is considered good and thus morally right and things that are bad or morally wrong. There are many different ethical theories and we cannot begin to explain them all in this introduction. However, you will recognize the three broad approaches outlined below in your own beliefs and culture and within professional organizations you work in.

 EXERCISE

Start by considering an action and think through how you might make an ethical decision: you are just about to deal with a situation with a person who needs your help; you have told them what you will do and when. Just at that moment, an emergency arises with another person. You are torn two ways: do you deal with the first person's needs or those of the second?

One way of viewing this is to concentrate on the immediate moment and the *action* you are about to take. This is rule-bound or 'duty' ethics and is familiar in many religious and other codes (Purlito, 2011). You have made a promise to the first person, which you will have to break if you do not return. This will affect their trust in you and the way you and your profession are viewed and respected. This approach is associated with the philosopher Immanuel Kant (1724–1804) who argued that people had a right to be treated with dignity and respect, and is called deontology, from the Greek word 'deonto' meaning 'duty'.

Another way of deciding what to do is to think of the *consequences* of your actions. What will be the outcome of your actions? Which person will suffer most if you neglect them? Which will benefit most from your time? If the emergency is a life-or-death situation, this is easy, but real-life practice is rarely that clear cut and you may have to weigh up which is the least bad, rather than best, outcome. The philosophers Jeremy Bentham (1748–1832) and John Stuart Mill (1806–73) are associated with the development of this thinking. It is called utilitarian or consequential ethics, where you try to calculate the action that will give the greatest good to the greatest number (Beauchamp & Childress, 2013; Purlito, 2011).

Finally you may find yourself thinking through all of these things, and on the basis of your *experience, knowledge and personal morality* you make what seems to be the wisest decision in this instance. This can be difficult to understand; think of someone (either a professional person, or maybe someone from your family or friends) who is the person you would go to if you were in trouble, whom you would trust to give you balanced, wise advice. In your professional life you wish to aspire to be as wise as they are, to develop the skills, knowledge and experience and become a respected expert in your field. This is called virtue ethics.

Where deontological and utilitarian ethics encourage you to think *What ought I to do?*, virtue ethics returns to the philosophical question *How ought I to be?* or *How should I live?* This links to the idea that caring, or the 'ethics of care', may have more personal meaning than objective rules regarding duty (Gilligan, Ward, McLean Taylor & Bardige, 1988). There are also parallels with 'values based practice' and reflection as discussed in medicine (Thornton, 2008), where ethically strong decision making ensures that 'good process' is seen to be as important as 'good outcome'.

 SEARCH AND EXPLORE

These ethical theories are complex and there is a great deal of information about them. Try searching on-line for the relevant words (for example 'virtue ethics' or 'deontology'); you will find simple, and more complex, explanations which may help you to analyse and think about your preferred approach.

Banks and Gallagher (2009) offer a useful explanation of how virtue ethics can work in health and social care. They trace its origins to ancient religions of China, Islam and Christianity, as well as to the Greek philosophers, particularly to Aristotle. Aristotle observed his society and tried to work out what was special about people who 'flourished' in their lives (Hursthouse, 1999). He identified that it was in their lifestyle, education and behaviour that they cultivated the 'cardinal' virtues of wisdom, courage, justice and temperance. Banks & Gallagher go on to suggest a wider set of virtues for the health and social care professions:

- care
- respectfulness

- trustworthiness
- justice
- courage
- integrity

A further and very important virtue is what they term 'professional wisdom' and is referred to by Aristotle and others as 'practical wisdom'. This is the essential skill of judgement:

- When is 'care' overbearing and cloying? When is it too casual, and thus not caring enough?
- When is rushing headlong into a situation appropriately courageous or wildly foolhardy?
- When is standing back wisely prudent or a cowardly cop-out?

Your professional wisdom is made up of your ability to understand, to perceive what is important; your 'moral imagination' (Banks & Gallagher, 2009, p. 85); and your reflective and decision making skills. We aim to help you to develop these important elements as you work through this book.

 TIME FOR REFLECTION

Returning to the example at the start of this section (where you were asked to imagine yourself faced with two competing actions: to deal with the first person's needs, whom you have already agreed to help, or the emergency that has just arisen), what approach would you choose?

As you can see, there is no single way to reflect on the ethics of professional practice, so the approach you choose to take is entirely yours, influenced by your upbringing, beliefs and personality. To us, the closest alignment with reflective practice is virtue ethics due to its harmony with professional values, its acknowledgement of an emotional, personal reaction to events, and its capacity to allow you to grow and change. Consequently, we will refer back to the virtues: care, respectfulness, trustworthiness, justice, courage and integrity on a number of occasions in this book to show how an appreciation of ethics and the development of professional wisdom may link to reflective practice.

 EXERCISE

We have deliberately presented our introduction to reflection as simply as possible in this chapter. If you are interested in taking a more detailed and critical look, we suggest that you start by going back to the seminal work:

1. Start with Schön's (1991) work and, having read chapter 2, explore in more detail by looking at later chapters where he adds more detailed justification. Do you agree with him? Do his ideas make sense to you?
2. There is a huge literature critiquing Schön's theories; do a literature search and find papers that are relevant to your area of professional practice – these will come in useful as you progress so the time will not be wasted! A published review that may help you get started is Mann, Gordon and MacLeod (2009).

Summary

Reflection asks you regularly to stop and think about what you are doing and why. The focus is on not only your own actions and feelings, but also the effect that you have on people you are responsible for and your fellow colleagues. In this chapter we have introduced you to the background to reflective practice; and to storytelling and ethics, two things we think are inseparable from reflection. In the next chapter, we will introduce you to some models of reflection, and from there we will begin to explore ways to express reflection, working alone and in groups, and some of the uses of, and challenges to, reflection.

Suggested reading for this chapter

Banks, S. & Gallagher, A. (2009). *Ethics in Professional Life: Virtues for Health and Social Care*. Basingstoke: Palgrave Macmillan.

This is a very good book explaining virtue ethics. It's readable if you just want to know a little bit more, but detailed and very well argued if you are interested in a more in-depth ethical argument.

Benner, P., Chesla, C. A. & Tanner, C. A. (2009). *Expertise in Nursing Practice: Caring, Clinical Judgement and Ethics* (2nd edn). New York: Springer Publishing Company.

Although written with nursing in mind, this is very interesting and important research that makes good links for you between ethics, professional practice and reflection. It also includes an explanation of Dreyfus and Dreyfus' model of skill acquisition.

Gilligan, C., Ward, J. V., McLean Taylor, J. & Bardige, B. (1988). *Mapping the Moral Domain: A Contribution of Woman's Thinking to Psychological Theory and Education.* Cambridge, MA: Harvard University Press.

This is serious theoretical work around the ethics of care and feminist ideas of moral reasoning. If you want to stretch yourself a bit, this is one we would recommend.

Purlito, R. (2011). *Ethical Dimensions in the Health Professions* (5th edn). Missouri: Elsevier Saunders Company.

There are many good texts on professional ethics, and you may already have a favourite. If not, this is a good one to start with.

Schön, D. A. (1991). *The Reflective Practitioner: How Professionals Think in Action.* Aldershot: Arena, Ashgate Publishing.

This is *the* seminal text on reflective practice – it's well worth looking at chapter 2, which will expand on the background in this chapter and is a good read.

CHAPTER TWO

The context of reflective practice: choosing an approach that works for you

---

Chapter Summary

In chapter 1, we introduced the idea of reflective practice, using Donald Schön's theories about reflection in and on action (Schön, 1991). Since this popularization of the concept, reflection has been absorbed into professional education and practice and a great deal has been written on the subject. There are now dozens of models and adaptations of models available for your use.

In this chapter we will explore in more detail the reasons why you might use reflective practice. We will do this by exploring various models and using stories. We offer some choices here and are sure that as a result of your reading and experience, you will be able to find those which suit you best.

Through studying this chapter and engaging in the exercises you will be able to:

- understand when and how to use reflection
- identify which model is of most use to you in a given situation
- develop the ability to create your own story for reflection

---

Why reflect?

Your first response to this may be that you are asked to – or even required to as part of a course you are undertaking. Once qualified, you may also be expected to keep a reflective portfolio as part of your continuing professional development. We believe that health and social care professions use reflective practice to:

- embed good practice
- record thinking processes
- develop skills
- improve practice
- move difficult situations forward

The reward for you as a professional is that this approach will make your practice more fulfilling and sustainable; it may also help you through a difficult or challenging time at work. Your reflective practice will improve the experience of people for whom you have responsibility and those you work with.

Embedding good practice
George tells you that he has slept better. And thanks you. Are you a miracle worker?

What happened? When you reflect on your previous visit to George, all you can see that you have done differently is to bring him his eye medication. Talking to George, he explains that, because he could see properly, he decided to do a bit of gardening. As the result of the gardening, he was properly hungry, he made himself a full supper, watched the late news and went to bed.

The small action of bringing the eye drops is good practice because of the impact it has had on George. Being able to see has led to him being able to exercise and eat properly, thus he was able to sleep. Having seen what has happened to George, you can understand that a small act can have disproportionately beneficial outcomes.

Recording thinking processes

How you think about your practice does not really matter; the key is to have a *record* of the process. This is common to almost all published models of reflection, some of which we outline later in this chapter, and use in the exercises we offer you. Your thinking may look messy and unfocused, it may not be in chronological order; but once you have captured it, you can begin to see a logical process.

Reflection does not have to be written, it could be an audio or pictorial record. Reflection other than written is discussed in detail in chapter 6. The important thing is that you can revisit it and reinterpret it when you need to, because it is through the process of this recording that you gain insight. It may help to apply a formal model to your reflections, but you may also choose to find your own route.

Developing skills

Knowledge is experiential; we learn through our successes and mistakes. Reflective practice helps us make the best of our experience and grow as a result. What you have learned from George is likely to have little to do with his ophthalmic condition, or the properties of the eye drops (this knowledge may or may not be part of your professional role). Likely to be more important are the listening and questioning skills you used when you were trying to understand why he was housebound, sad and listless. When you analyse the incident into its component parts, the skill of listening is highlighted. The next time that you are faced with a situation like this or a situation in your own professional role where you actively listen to what a person is saying about their life, the likelihood is that you will be able to make a positive intervention earlier.

Improve practice

Reflection has the potential to improve practice – for example, it may make you more open to learning and responsive to others; the evidence base for this is discussed in more detail in chapter 9. Critical Incident Technique, which is used extensively in reflective practice and is described in more detail later in this chapter, was specifically developed in the 1950s by Flanagan to help aeroplane pilots to reflect on successes and near-misses, explicitly to help them improve their performance, with life-saving consequences (Ghaye & Lillyman, 2006). A systematic search of the literature suggests there is some empirical evidence in medicine and health care to support the role of reflection in improving practice (Mann et al., 2009). In addition, earlier research by Martha MacLeod on the practice of busy, experienced surgical ward sisters identified their openness to learning and a reflective approach as key factors in their successful practice (MacLeod, 1996). For social work, Brookfield argues strongly for the centrality of 'critical' reflection to practice (Brookfield, 2009). Whatever your motivation, reflection gives you a framework on which you can build further learning. Often, during reflective practice, you will see where your best skills lie and recognize that you have capabilities you hadn't expected.

Move difficult situations forward
When things go wrong, reflective practice can help you to identify where a change or intervention could have improved the outcome for all of those involved. When a tragedy happens, everyone wants somebody to blame and fingers are quickly pointed. Reflective practice takes the heat out of the situation and gives you a safe process in which to explore your role and involvement. It may help you isolate a moment that you had not remembered under pressure. Perhaps there are signs that you missed because you were stressed or something that you understood in one way was meant in another. By breaking things up into their component pieces, it becomes easier to identify gaps and omissions.

Reflection can also help you to accept when you have failed. There is no health or social care professional who has not made a mistake. But recognizing small mistakes for what they are can prevent us making bigger ones at a later stage. We learn not to take complicated decisions when we are tired, or to stand back from situations that we simply cannot handle at that moment. As we develop our professionalism, we understand that it is not a sign of weakness to say that there are times when we cannot cope; we have a responsibility to ourselves as well as the people with whom we work. Sometimes the most professional thing you can do is hand over to somebody else. The importance of reflection when things go wrong is explored in detail in chapter 7.

How to reflect?

We hope we have convinced you that reflection is a worthwhile activity. In your everyday practice and as part of a course, it is a useful way to expand your learning and make the links between theory and practice. There are many approaches in the literature, generally referred to as models of reflection, so a little explanation of 'models' may be helpful.

The word 'model' has many meanings. A person strutting down the catwalk 'models' clothes, showing the audience how the outfit looks; this illustrates that 'model' can mean an idealized or perfect version of something. A model may also be a replica – many toys are models: cars, dolls, aeroplanes and soft toys make no claim to be the 'real thing' but are very important in play, allowing children to explore and experiment with concepts within the real world. Replicas, however, are not always toys: an engineer may make a very precise or computer-generated model in order to investigate and predict likely outcomes in a safe and controlled way.

Models may also be conceptual. This is where we envision the way something should be, an idealized state. Such models are often so embedded into our cultural outlook and education that we struggle to 'see' them, but they are all around! To illustrate this point we will use a conceptual model that is recognizable (but not necessarily the same) in all human societies.

 TIME FOR REFLECTION

'Family': stop for a moment and reflect about what your idea of a family is . . . got it? – right, read on –

A recognizable 'idealized' view of the family is of a 'nuclear family' said to consist of a male and female adult and their genetic offspring and an 'extended family' which includes other relatives such as grandparents, aunts, uncles and cousins (Macionis, 2010). How does this match with your thoughts above? There is a fair chance that you recognize this model, but that it does not necessarily represent the 'family' to which you belong. Many children live with one parent, or with adults and other children to whom they are not biologically linked. The 'nuclear' model is challenged by equality legislation that demands the recognition of same-sex partnerships, of single parents, of equal responsibility shared by mothers and fathers, and much more. Although research shows that views of the family vary (Hakim, 2003), the nuclear family model is nevertheless recognizable and used as a benchmark against which to evaluate relationships and child rearing.

Perhaps you have a more abstract view of family? It may be that it is a state of mind, or is manifested in the way a group of people interact and support each other. Thus a group of people sharing a house may support each other financially and emotionally, forming a 'family group' with very few of the biological relationships above in place. These may be what are called 'families of affinity' (Macionis, 2010, p. 463). Would you say this is also a 'model' family, or is it something else? Whatever your view, the concept 'family' is well recognized and allows for comparisons and for shared understanding.

Models of reflection are conceptual too – like 'family', they offer a structure that can be examined, followed, challenged and critiqued. You may find one useful to help you to get your own thoughts into order, to deal with an issue that is emotionally upsetting or to plan a piece of reflective writing.

Choosing an approach that works for you

We have thought a lot about how to advise you on reflective models; there are so many! In order to make sense of this, firstly we ask you to contemplate the ways in which you learn – what helps and hinders you to learn? Do you think in words, pictures or music? Do you prefer to learn in a quiet room, or are you at your best walking around? We will also offer you a top ten of models to help you to find one you think you could work with, or will match your needs. We will then detail a few approaches that we draw on regularly in this book. However, perhaps most importantly, we will encourage you to contemplate your own model.

Learning styles
The literature on learning styles says that we all tend to have a preferred way of learning (Tileston, 2005). Some literature describes people as 'reflectors', 'pragmatists', 'activists' or 'theorists' (Honey & Mumford, 1992). Others suggest that people learn best by 'seeing', or 'doing', or 'hearing' (Fleming, 2001) (see table 2.1).

 SEARCH AND EXPLORE

If you are curious to know what your preferred learning style is just type 'learning style questionnaire' into any search engine and you will find many free surveys that you can use to explore your own style.

Your self-awareness or a learning style questionnaire may have shown you to be reflective, or to learn best by thinking or drawing; this may influence the model you choose. However,

Table 2.1 Learning styles (adapted from Fleming, 2001; Honey & Mumford, 1992)

	Auditory learners 'hear'		
V			Read/
I			
S	Pragmatist – 'does'	Activist – 'feels'	write
U			
A			learners
L			
			do
Learners	Theorist – 'conceptualizes'	Reflector – 'evaluates'	
			just
'see'			that
	Kinaesthetic learners 'get their hands dirty'		

remain open to trying new styles, rather than being restricted by the style you are most familiar with. There is a growing body of evidence that challenges the validity of individual learning styles (Harold, Mark, Doug & Robert, 2008; Sanderson, 2011) and further evidence that, even when we have preferences, this does not necessarily mean we learn more effectively (Koonce, Giuse & Storrow, 2011). Just because 'reflector' may not be your strongest style, that does not mean that you cannot learn, or develop reflective skills.

Top ten models

In order to illustrate our point about learning styles, we are going to present the top ten as a written list, as a picture and as a quick-view table.

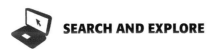 **SEARCH AND EXPLORE**

We have given at least one key reference for each of the models, so that you have an academic starting point, but you will also find that there is material about each of them on the internet. Watch out though – you will find that older versions can be confusing, so look for the dates!

The top ten list (in no particular order)

(1) Bolton believes the act of writing down a reflection is itself part of the process of developing the reflection (Bolton, 2010). She describes her model as 'through the mirror' writing, using Lewis Carroll's *Alice Through the Looking Glass* as a metaphor. The mirror permits us to, or even demands that we, look at the world very differently, and in doing so it reveals unexpected aspects of our understanding and practice. She describes reflection in action as 'a hawk in the mind constantly circling, watching and advising on practice' (p. 33). The model asks you to write and re-write a reflection, progressively developing your reflection alone, and with the help of a trusted reader. Doing this is remarkably powerful and you may be surprised at what you produce. It takes a little time and effort to do this, but if writing is a medium you want to use, it's well worth the effort. In addition, if you are teaching reflection, this may offer you a safe and trustworthy structure.

(2) Moon's work on keeping a reflective learning journal or diary is more a learning guide than a single model (Moon, 2006). As the reason for keeping a journal will vary, she offers a range of suggestions, techniques and exercises to get the most out of the learning experience. Well worth exploring if keeping a journal is something you want, or are required, to do. It is also useful for teaching.

(3) Schön's ladder of reflection is a technique to use with a coach (Schön, 1991). The coach may demonstrate, critique, reflect and question, whilst the student observes, reflects, imitates and develops their own practice. The aim is to improve the student's practice, and to strengthen their confidence and skill. This is intended to be an active approach, with dialogue and movement, not sitting down to talk or write. It is described by Schön for use with

architects and musicians, but would work well with any 'performance', such as managing a difficult meeting or performing a skill.

(4) Gibbs' reflective cycle (Gibbs, 1988) is cited in many reflective practice texts (Bulman & Schutz, 2008; Ghaye & Lillyman, 2006). It uses a cyclical set of questions to guide you through thinking about what happened, your thoughts, feelings, analysis and actions. The advantage of this model is its straightforwardness: the questions are not difficult and can be easily applied in more or less any setting. You could use this to reflect alone quietly, to structure an entry in a reflective journal, or to talk through an issue with colleagues or a supervisor. A further advantage is that it includes evaluation and action planning. It is generally not enough just to review a situation; you will want to learn from this and apply that learning in the future. However, it can be used in a very superficial way – it's up to you to develop it, so it may not really push you to think critically about your practice, or to grow confident in reflective writing.

(5) Mezirow has developed a model of reflection over many decades. He believes that critical reflection can be the trigger to 'transformative learning', which is discussed in detail in chapter 1 of his 1990 book (Mezirow, 1990). Reflection is a form of thinking, but is more than *just* thinking. By assessment of the assumptions on which our thoughts and decisions are based, we can really critique what we do. Thus he is concerned to make us confront the background to our actions, as a way of accessing transformative learning – this he considers to be a very important learning act. It is not a model for the faint-hearted, or for a brief dipping of your toes in the water. It is complex and demanding so you may be put off by the dense language and by the many versions as it has developed and changed over time. However, it is probably the most cerebral of the models, so if thinking deeply is something you

feel you need or want to do, you may come to find its promise of transforming your learning an addictive choice.

(6) Johns' model of reflection was designed as an educational tool for nurses learning reflective practice (Johns, 2009), but if you are not a nurse do not be put off – the technique is pretty universal. The model asks the reflector a series of cue and supplementary questions that explore the focus of the reflection, analysis and learning. The question-and-answer format lends itself to supervision, or at least dialogue with one other person, but the detailed structure also means that you can quite effectively use the model on your own. Therefore it has the potential to be used to structure a reflective essay or journal entry and may be very helpful, particularly if you are unsure about reflective writing and want some help, or you are a teacher supporting your students. However, its linear, detailed questioning technique may stifle free-thinking reflection.

(7) Fook and Gardner advocate critical reflection in a group reflective setting where description, reflective questioning and re-thinking theory are important stages (Fook & Gardner, 2007). It is unusual to find a model that actively encourages group discussion, rather than personal introspection or coach/student, supervisor/supervisee relationships. It is also one of the models, like Mezirow's, that very deliberately pushes the reflector to look beyond themselves and the current situation and to critique the underlying assumptions and constructs. Not one for a beginner to tackle on their own, but a good and challenging option, with great potential as an aid to anyone wanting help with facilitating group reflection.

(8) A simplification of reflection to three cue questions – 'What? So what? Now what?' – was first published in 1970 (Borton, 1970), but the model has since been picked up by several other writers (Driscoll, 2000; Rolfe, Jasper &

Freshwater, 2011). Driscoll uses it in supervision and, like those of Gibbs and Johns, the model offers a processed series of questions. We think this is the most universal and useful description of this type of model: simple enough for a quick individual reflection but flexible enough to scaffold an essay, a diary entry, blog or group reflection as well as supervision. This is one of our preferred approaches and is described in more detail later in this chapter.

(9) Flanagan's Critical Incident Technique, also one of our preferred approaches, is not exactly a reflective model, but is so versatile and well used it is one of the techniques examined in more detail below. The aim is to deconstruct an incident in which an intervention has made a difference, to use this to identify good and bad practice and thus improve performance. The technique could be individual, collective, verbal, written, a one-off or a series . . . thus it is useful in a lot of different circumstances.

(10) Finally, we want to offer you our Reflective Timeline: not a model, more a way of thinking we have developed through talking about, and writing, this book. The full outline is provided later in the chapter; it was born out of the ways in which we described reflection to each other, and our wish to move away from cyclical models in which professionals can get stuck and struggle to move on. It has sufficient structure to help in putting a reflection together, but is fluid and flexible.

 SEARCH AND EXPLORE

All of the models mentioned in the clouds in figure 2.1, except for the Reflective Timeline, can be found on the internet – type in some detail and have a look for yourself.

The top ten picture

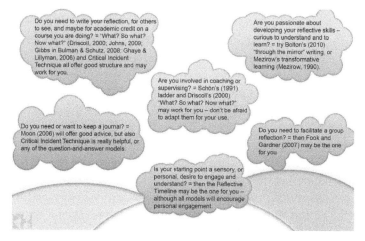

Do you need to write your reflection, for others to see, and maybe for academic credit on a course you are doing? = 'What? So what? Now what?' (Driscoll, 2000; Johns, 2009; Gibbs in Bulman & Schutz, 2008; Ghaye & Lillyman, 2006) and Critical Incident Technique all offer good structure and may work for you.

Are you passionate about developing your reflective skills – curious to understand and to learn? = try Bolton's (2010) 'through the mirror' writing, or Mezirow's transformative learning (Mezirow, 1990).

Are you involved in coaching or supervising? = Schön's (1991) ladder and Driscoll's (2000) 'What? So what? Now what?' may work for you – don't be afraid to adapt them for your use.

Do you need or want to keep a journal? = Moon (2006) will offer good advice, but also Critical Incident Technique is really helpful, or any of the question-and-answer models.

Do you need to facilitate a group reflection? = then Fook and Gardner (2007) may be the one for you

Is your starting point a sensory, or personal, desire to engage and understand? = then the Reflective Timeline may be the one for you – although all models will encourage personal engagement.

Figure 2.1 The top ten picture

The top ten quick-view table

Model	Writing	Thinking	Group	1:1
Table 2.2 The top ten quick-view list				
'What? So what? Now what?' (Driscoll, 2000)	☺	☺	☺	☺
Gibbs' reflective cycle (Ghaye & Lillyman, 2006; Gibbs, 1988)	☺	☺	☺	
Through the mirror reflection (Bolton, 2010)	☺	☺		☺
Schön's ladder of reflection (Schön, 1991)		☺		☺
Johns' reflective cycle (Johns, 2009)	☺	☺		☺
Critical Incident Technique	☺	☺	☺	☺
Mezirow's perspective transformation (Mezirow, 1990)	☺	☺		☺
Reflecting in a journal (Moon, 2006)	☺	☺		
Critical group reflection (Fook & Gardner, 2007)		☺	☺	
The Reflective Timeline	☺	☺	☺	☺

One further model, that is not in our top ten but we think is worth exploring, is a visual model called KAWA developed in Japan for occupational therapy (Iwama, 2006). Taking a river as a metaphor, it encourages the user to think about the barriers and enablers to reflection at a point in their development. By building up a picture of your river, you can explore pictorially rather than in writing. This model is discussed a lot on the internet, so it's worth browsing if you think it sounds interesting, and it will be discussed in more detail in chapter 6, where we look at reflecting in other ways.

Our preferred approaches

The Reflective Timeline
Mirror, mirror on the wall . . .

One of our criticisms of many published models is their emphasis on a cyclical process. This can lead you to think that you are never going to escape from the reflection you are doing and therefore nothing changes. But to build professional expertise it is essential to understand when to move on, taking your knowledge with you. We have all said about someone who has gone back and back over an incident, 'You need to move on.'

Think of a mirror. None of us look at our reflection in a mirror to make sure we remain the same. We want to see what can be made better. Perhaps our hair needs brushing or our shirt isn't straight or we have another wrinkle. The first two are easy to remedy, and perhaps that wrinkle disappears when we smile. But at some point we all have to turn away from the mirror and face the world.

Starting from the stages of reflection (Schön, 1991), the process we have used to model our thinking throughout this book and for our own reflective practice when working together can be summed up as:

In the moment
Looking back

Looking again
Moving on

In the moment is the start of the process. It is not a neutral or zero point. It is influenced by the world around you, what you know, whom you are working with and the whole complicated and unique bag of culture, fears and feelings that makes you 'you'.

Looking back is when you analyse the situation on which you are reflecting. It is like looking at a wall of blocks and breaking it up into pieces. This is when you might think 'Why was I feeling like that?' and recognize that, because the milk was off, you had not had your usual cup of tea.

Looking again takes those pieces and makes a careful examination of them before re-assembling them. This time the wall may be longer or wider or even the same, but the same pieces may not be in the same order.

Moving on is the point when what you have reflected on leads you to a moment of enlightenment, giving you the energy and impulse to do things differently. The way in which you move on may involve changing aspects of poor practice, leaving behind personal worries, accepting responsibility. It could be as simple as realizing that, in the circumstances, you did your best – which is really not a simple process at all.

We will illustrate the use of the Reflective Timeline in chapter 3.

'What? So what? Now what?'
If you are more of a list person, or like more structure, then this version of the model developed to aid clinical supervision may work for you (Driscoll, 2000). On the surface, this model is as simple as it sounds. Thus *What?* asks you to describe what you think is happening, what you understand from the situation. Then you ask *So what?* – a 'why' question that encourages

analysis and evaluation; and the *Now what?* where you apply what you know to deciding what to do next. Driscoll expands on these simple questions with a series of more detailed cues, in which he asks:

WHAT? *(description)*
- What is the purpose of returning to the situation?
- What happened?
- What did I see/do?
- What was my reaction to it?
- What did other people do who were involved in this?

SO WHAT? *(analysis)*
- How did I feel at the time of the event?
- Were those feelings I had any different from those of other people who were also involved at the time?
- Are my feelings now, after the event, any different from what I experienced at the time?
- Do I still feel troubled – if so, in what way?
- What were the effects of what I did (or did not do)?
- What positive effects emerge now for me from the event that happened in practice?
- What have I noticed about my behaviour and practice by taking a more measured look at it?
- How can observations from others on the way I acted at the time help me to reflect?

NOW WHAT? *(action)*
- What are the implications for me and others based on my description and analysis?
- What difference does it make if I choose to do nothing?
- Where can I get more information to help me manage a similar situation again?
- How can I modify my practice for the future?
- What help do I need to help me 'action' the results of my reflections?
- Which aspect should be tackled first?
- How will I notice that I am any different in practice?

- What is the main learning I take from my reflection on my practice?

(adapted from Driscoll, 2000, p. 28)

Designed to aid supervision, the model works particularly well as a personal contemplation or in a dialogue with a colleague or supervisor. This very personal focus ('How did *I* come across? What behaviour did *I* use / could *I* change?') may not push you to look at the wider policy, political and social factors that might be affecting practice, but don't let this put you off trying it. It can be used very successfully to structure your thoughts and to construct a piece of written reflection. If 'we' is substituted for 'I', it can also form a useful basis for group supervision.

Critical Incident Technique

The third structure we want to offer was not developed for reflective practice as we now define it, but has been used in a wide variety of professions and in research for around sixty years, so is well worth trying.

Flanagan first published a report on its use in 1954, although it had been researched for some decades before that. Flanagan used it to analyse successful and unsuccessful missions for air force pilots in the USA in World War Two. Since then, it has been used extensively in research and in professional education (Benner et al., 2009; Bulman & Schutz, 2008; Butterfield, Amundson, Maglio & Borgen, 2005). The basic stages of Critical Incident Technique are as follows:

(1) Identify an incident that is 'critical' for you – this will be an occasion when your actions made a difference (positively or negatively) to the outcome of an aspect of your practice. Your incidents can be as open as your imagination or situation allows, from an individual event through to a research project in which you ask many people to complete the process and analyse the results.

(2) Try to describe what is critical about this incident for you

in as much detail as you can, and as is necessary for your purpose. Draw it, create a timeline, record your memory of it – whatever way works best for you.

(3) Now get down to some analysis – ask yourself:
- Why is this critical?
- What are the key components of the incident?

(4) What conclusions can you draw from this? What theories or research can you bring to bear to help you understand what is happening? This is an opportunity to review the situation critically – ask questions such as:
- Can I see how my theoretical knowledge applies to this incident?
- Does this support or challenge my professional understanding?
- What gaps are there in my knowledge, understanding and skills that I could work on?

(5) And finally, what does your critical analysis suggest should be done differently, or should change?

Critical Incident Technique is very flexible: you could analyse an incident that is highly personal; an incident that involved a number of people, for whom it is critical in different ways; incidents on the level of a whole organization, or in relation to policy. All can be successfully explored using this model.

DIY reflection

But do remember – the reflection is yours, and you can do it any way you like. Don't be frightened to abandon all ideas about preferred learning styles, lists of questions and predetermined processes. The famous fictional detective Sherlock Holmes talks of 'two pipe solutions': when faced with a particularly difficult challenge, he needed to contemplate through the duration of two whole pipes of his favourite smoke to reach a conclusion. This cannot be rushed. You will have your own versions of

Holmes's two pipes – a walk or run in the park, a long bath, a chat with a trusted friend, pen and paper, your laptop . . .

You might want to ask yourself why you are reflecting, and recall the five reasons we offered at the start of the chapter – to:

- embed good practice
- record thinking processes
- develop skills
- improve practice
- move difficult situations forward

But above all, have belief in your own ability and do it in a way that works for you.

Limitations of models

Though models have a lot to offer, you can get bogged down trying to fulfil the model rather than focusing on the issue. Models come up with neat solutions and we can find ourselves trying to model the model instead of moving forward towards our own solution.

All models are hypothetical and, though they are created to mirror reality, real life is more complicated. Something goes wrong at work the same day as you fail an exam and the car gets a flat tyre. No amount of modelling can address this and your feelings.

Different models have been written from particular approaches such as social work, education or health. In multi-agency work, each professional perspective, though valid for that profession, may be unhelpful when several practitioners are working together, especially if they come from different cultural backgrounds.

Some models expect you to reflect using a particular medium, for example keeping a reflective note book. This might not be possible in your area of practice because of con-fidentiality, or it may not suit your preferred learning style. Many reflective models say you cannot reflect in isolation but you may not have anyone you can share your reflection with. Increasingly, digital media are being used to record and share reflection, on mobile devices, through digital stories and in blogs, wikis and portfolios (Brown, 2010; Gardner, Bridges & Walmsley, 2012; Lai & Calandra, 2010; Montgomery, 2003). A review of some current ideas and developments is included in chapter 6.

Sometimes it is possible to isolate your professional self from your personal self; although this can help with some reflection, it is a limited approach because reflection stems from one's life experience and you may not be able to see your own prejudices and gaps in your knowledge. Our own culture and background, as well as our perceptions of others, are part of the thinking process we bring to reflection.

A dependence on models and their outcomes can stop you moving on and developing your own solutions. The time to move on from a model might be when:

- it is no longer challenging you
- there are things you need to think through that the model doesn't address
- you are spending more time analysing the model than the problem
- you've made a decision
- you have changed your practice

Limitations may also be much more than just getting stuck in a model that does not work for you. Reflection can be a Pandora's Box from which fear of personal disclosure, tensions with other colleagues, legal and ethical dilemmas all come rushing out when you raise the lid. These difficulties are dealt with later in chapters 7 and 8.

Using stories for reflection

Stories are powerful things. You will know from reading this book that we believe that stories can be used to promote reflection. Every time you send a text, tweet or email about something you have done or seen, you are telling part of a story. Stories are one of the ways that we find common purpose with other people, and this is true for all cultures.

You will have been taught at school that all stories have beginnings, middles and ends. From watching soap operas or television series, you will be aware of how frustrating it can be to miss the end of the story because you will already have created a likely outcome for your favourite characters and want to know if that was the resolution of their story. The examples we use in this book interrupt the story and ask for your response at different points in the tale. We have made up the examples so that they fit the tasks we are asking you to perform to enhance your reflective practice. In some of them we have used our own experience, while taking care to protect the anonymity of those involved; in others we have thought up situations in order to challenge you as the reader.

Stories used for reflection need to be as open as possible. This means the people reflecting on them can interpret what is happening from a number of professional viewpoints. But they also need to be detailed.

For example, *Geoff has problems accessing his front door from the street* tells us that a man called Geoff finds it difficult to get into his home from the road. It does not tell us whether the problem is to do with Geoff and his health or with a different access problem, perhaps local children calling him names because he has a mental health problem.

So let us expand the example a little: *Geoff, who suffers from Parkinson's, has problems accessing his front door from the street. There are seven steps to the front door.*

We now know a little more. This more detailed example tells us the nature of Geoff's problem and we know that, because of his illness, he has mobility problems. We can now visualize that there are steps, but not whether they go up or down to the front door. Perhaps you are thinking that what Geoff needs is a handrail to solve the problem, but what if we add a stick?

*Geoff has Parkinson's, walks with a stick and has problems
accessing his front door from the street. There are seven steps up
to the door and when Geoff returns from doing his shopping he
finds it impossible to climb the steps with his stick and shopping
at the same time.*

We now have a clear picture of Geoff and his difficulties.
You will notice that we have not described him or where he
lives as they are not relevant to the current story we are creating for reflection. In your mind you have probably visualized a
front door, but the actual nature of the door is not relevant and
therefore the story does not describe it. But what your mind
has done is fill in details of the story. In this way you have
helped to place Geoff in a world that you can explore in more
detail while you reflect on his problems.

In this book we have given names to the characters
involved. Some examples you will have come across in other
contexts will, in keeping with patient confidentiality, have
described the people involved in reflective stories as 'Client
Y' or 'Patient Z'. We prefer to give those involved names, but
are aware that names carry certain values. Names in most
cultures are class-, age-, sex- and race-specific. When you
hear a name, you make judgements about the owner of that
name. We are aware of this, but since it is something you will
encounter in your own practice, we have chosen to give our
characters names.

Where necessary, we have given background to the characters we have created, but in Nilam's story in chapter 3 we
have only described her family life after we have given you the
critical incident in the story, which is the teacher's discovery
of the burn on her leg. If the teacher had not noticed the mark,
Nilam's life would have gone on very much as it had before. So
it is important to decide where your story begins, and at what
point you want others to begin their reflection on it.

You do not always need to create a new story for reflection.
We have had some interesting discussions when we have

used traditional stories as a basis for group reflection about inter-agency working. For example, the story of Little Red Riding Hood who went to visit her grandmother and discovered she had been eaten by a wolf opened the door to child protection issues, lifting and handling, the grandmother's diet and the rights of wolves. Using a shared, familiar story can be a very positive way into inter-agency working.

The great thing about stories for reflection is they don't have to be fully formed. You don't have to tie up all the loose ends to produce some form of satisfactory solution and what your teachers would call a conclusion. If you have explored and examined ideas and possible outcomes of a certain situation, the story you have created has done its work. It has shown you a way forward.

 TIME FOR REFLECTION

We have introduced a lot of different ideas and models in this chapter. Take a moment to reflect on which you find most useful or interesting. There will be many opportunities over the remaining chapters to put them into use.

 EXERCISE

We have introduced a number of models in this chapter, with thumbnail sketches of how they work and how you might use them. Some involve more complex language and ideas, but in all cases the level of reflection and criticality will rest with you. If you want to test yourself out, and you are prepared to give some time to writing:

Get hold of Bolton's (2010) work (or search for her work on the internet). Use her 'through the mirror' technique. You will need to be prepared to work on a draft, to re-draft and to share your work with at least one person who can offer you feedback. Approach this with an open mind and you will find that you have written something with more detail and depth than you would have predicted at the start. You may surprise yourself, or be surprised by the feedback you get from your reader, who maybe sees things in the writing that you were unaware of.

Summary

We have now given you some background on the use of models in reflective practice, and introduced you to some of the many types that are already available. Models are not all there is to reflection but may help you to get started, particularly if reflection does not come naturally to you, or if you have to write your reflection and want something that will help you to do a good job.

We will expand on this in the next two chapters, looking at the timeline for reflection in chapter 3 and at writing for reflection in chapter 4.

Suggested reading for this chapter

Bulman, C. & Schutz, S. (2008). *Reflective Practice in Nursing.* Oxford: Blackwell.

This is a very useful, all-round book about reflective practice. The critical and comprehensive review of the literature is particularly good, and useful regardless of your professional background.

Driscoll, J. (2000). *Practising Clinical Supervision.* London: Bailliere Tindall.

A useful and well-written 'how to' book for supervision. If you like the 'What? So what? Now what?', it's a good place to start to develop your understanding.

Ghaye, T. & Lillyman, S. (2006). *Learning and Critical Incidents: Reflective Practice for Health Care Professionals* (2nd edn). Salisbury: Mark Allen Publishing.

A good, fairly simple résumé of many models, a useful reference and starting point.

Mezirow, J. (1990). *Fostering Critical Reflection in Adulthood: A Guide to Transformative and Emancipatory Learning.* San Francisco: Jossey-Bass.

If you really want to get into Mezirow, I would recommend having a go at this version – but it is not an easy read.

Moon, J. A. (2006). *Learning Journals: A Handbook for Reflective Practice and Professional Development.* Abingdon: Routledge.

A good text for understanding reflective journals – quite theoretical and well referenced, so useful academically.

CHAPTER THREE

The Reflective Timeline

Chapter Summary

In chapters 1 and 2, we have introduced you to our ideas about what becoming a reflective practitioner is about, and to some of the models and theory that may help you on your journey. In this chapter, we show you how the Reflective Timeline works. You will see how your professionalism is one of the steps on a journey that involves others, illustrating the importance of professional and inter-professional working. You will understand where your involvement starts and where it ends.

Through studying this chapter and engaging in the exercises, you will be able to:

- locate your own profession within the wider context of your role
- recognize the importance of each stage along the timeline
- reflect on your own timelines in a given situation

In any Reflective Timeline there are many different professionals involved at each stage. For example, in the story that unfolds in this chapter, the timeline starts with a school-teacher; however, a midwife, a family doctor, a social worker and a children's nurse are just some of the people who are also part of this timeline. Many other professionals will be part of any care or support that you give. Each professional involved comes from a different perspective and has a different set of skills, but you will all share similar professional values.

Being a professional

You will have noticed that we use the word 'professional' frequently in this book and regularly ask you to be aware of and respect the professional role of others, so it is worth taking a few moments to think about what this might mean.

 TIME FOR REFLECTION

Stop and think for a moment: identify someone you know whom you would describe as a 'professional'. Ask yourself what it is that makes them a professional and jot down these key features.

In common language we use the word 'professional' in many different ways, so it does not have a clear definition. In boxing and many other sports, someone may be professional or amateur. Both could be equally skilled and respected in their field; the difference in title reflects whether they are paid or not. In other circumstances, 'profession' may be contrasted to 'vocation'. 'Vocation' has religious connotations, and is strongly associated historically with some health professions such as medicine and nursing, with doing social work and with religious duty. However, in contemporary language it has a different meaning. 'Vocational' qualifications usually refer to courses leading to employment that have a practical or applied element. 'Vocation' may be associated with lower pay, or with voluntary unpaid work, adding another confusing dimension.

The academic literature does not really clarify these definitions. Van Mook looked at assessing professionalism in medical students, putting the emphasis on professional behaviour rather than personality traits, and relating this to ethical reasoning and behaviour (van Mook, van Luijk, O'Sullivan,

Wass, Schuwirth & van der Vleuten, 2009). Further research (Rogers & Ballantyne, 2010) adds the capacity for reflection to the attributes. This approach is used in chapter 7 where we discuss reflection and ethical practice, particularly where there are difficult decisions to be made, and where you, the professional, may have made a mistake.

Further research with dental students used eight 'professional attributes' to analyse professionalism (Pau & Croucher, 2003, p. 124):

- Ability to recognize personal/professional strengths and limitations
- Ability to listen attentively
- Caring and compassionate nature
- Spirit of curiosity
- Unprejudiced respect for others transcending gender, culture, background, etc.
- Ability to cope with stress, uncertainty and setback
- Commitment to manage your own learning
- Ability to communicate effectively with each other

For others, for example Litchfield, Frawley and Nettleton (2010), the emphasis is on being 'work ready', and although there are some overlaps, particularly regarding communication, their list is different (p. 521):

- Ethics and professionalism
- A global perspective
- Communication capacity
- Ability to work well in a team
- Ability to apply knowledge
- Creative problem solving and critical thinking skills

As you can see, both of these sets of attributes also link closely to ethical practice, and have overlaps with the virtues identified in chapter 1 (Banks & Gallagher, 2009).

These studies provide just a small example of the many different definitions in use. They represent a move away from a vocational ethos towards skilled, highly employable, reflective, ethically aware individuals.

Working inter-professionally

EXERCISE

In the section above, we asked you to identify someone whom you thought of as 'professional', and we identified a number of shared attributes, regardless of which profession you or they may practise. What we would like you to do now is to think about all of the professionals who interact with your role. Try focusing on a client, patient or service user with whom you have had contact – someone whom you needed to support or help professionally. Focusing on that person, and what you know about their lives, make a list of all the professions he or she is likely to have encountered over the last few weeks.

We identified Francis, who is depressed following a cardiovascular accident.

The definitions of 'professional' identified at the start of this chapter all relate to *individual* people; training for your profession will include specific knowledge and skills that make you, for example, a social worker, dentist, doctor, allied health professional or nurse. However, it is rare for any health or social care professional to work in isolation, as the focus of our roles is usually the health or wellbeing of individuals, who will have contact with many professionals. It is equally rare for an individual's care or support to be managed by a single, isolated professional.

The World Health Organization published a far-reaching report on inter-professional education and collaboration (WHO, 2010), which is a worthwhile read for any professional interested in the wellbeing of the population. Whilst global catastrophes, war and famine may seem a long way from your own area of practice, the message that inter-professional collaboration is essential is hard to dispute. Interestingly, the difficulties that health and social care professionals seem

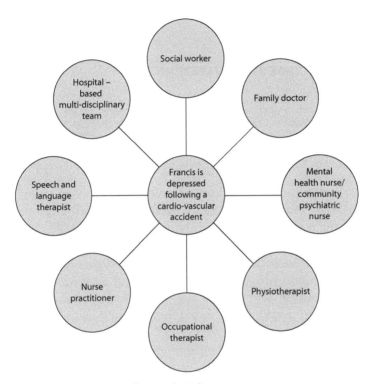

Figure 3.1 An inter-professional circle

to have in working together are not always recognized in other sectors. A refreshing perspective in the cultural industries is about working together creatively, rather than being embroiled in differences and in professional 'politics' (David, 2011).

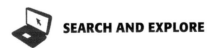 **SEARCH AND EXPLORE**

There is a huge body of literature on inter-professional learning and education. Try searching for the 'Centre for the Advancement of Interprofessional Education CAIPE'. Look on websites from your profession, or national organizations such as the 'Higher Education Academy', and you will find reports, reviews of the literature, research, special interest groups and much more.

Shared values

TIME FOR REFLECTION

At the beginning of this chapter, we asked you to consider the key features of being a professional. How closely do they match with what you have read so far? Do you think your profession is similar to, or very different from, other professions? Look back on your list. Do you want to modify it? Have we missed something that is important to you?

Factors included in all of our professional codes and standards of ethics are likely to be respect for others, a primary focus on the person or people for whom you are responsible rather than yourself, the ability to suspend personal judgement, and the ability to work collectively, even with people you may not like or agree with, towards a common goal. In practice these standards are hard to meet and we will explore these issues further in chapters 7 and 8, but they should be at the heart of your professionalism.

This chapter in particular shows how each Reflective Timeline can be seen in relation to others.

Nilam's Day

When Nilam, ten, is getting changed for sport, her teacher Mr Parker notices that she has a burn on her leg. When he asks Nilam what has happened, she says that she was trying to iron her skirt while she was wearing it and got the iron too hot. The teacher asked why she was ironing her skirt when she was wearing it. Nilam explains she was in a hurry to get her younger siblings, aged six and two, dressed because her mother is ill and couldn't get out of bed.

TIME FOR REFLECTION

From your professional perspective, what is the first thing in the story that jumps out at you?

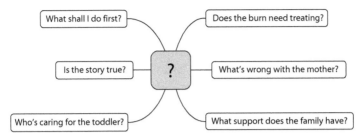

Figure 3.2 First thoughts

Your initial response to this will depend on your background and training. For example, if you have ever been too ill to care physically for your children, you will know how frightening that is. If you have been a young carer like Nilam, you will know how torn you are between the need for help and loyalty to your family. If you have ever had contact with a two-year-old, you will know how much energy they have. Even if you doubt the story, the evidence is there: Nilam has the mark of the iron on her leg.

Depending on your area of expertise, your primary concern may be anything from treating the burn to your legal responsibilities for safeguarding children.

 TIME FOR REFLECTION

Thinking about the story again, what are your perceptions now? Do you have questions you want to ask? What are they? Have they changed? If they have, you are already practising reflection.

The Reflective Timeline

All reflection has a timeline to it. We suggest that this is likely to fall into four categories:

In the → looking → looking → moving on
moment   back   again

Using Nilam's story as an example, we will now explore the Reflective Timeline in more detail. This begins at the point where awareness is raised. In this case, it begins when the teacher notices the burn on Nilam's leg. We have chosen to start the timeline at Nilam's school to show you that reflection is important for all professionals and that a timeline for you, in social work or in health, is likely to exist for other professionals as well. An allied health professional, nurse, midwife, family doctor or social worker in contact with Nilam, her siblings or her mother will have had different starting points for engagement with the family. An emergency happens to be the trigger in this timeline, but it could equally well be something with positive implications.

▶▶ *In the moment*

This is the moment, when working with Nilam, that your professionalism takes over and you make immediate decisions. It is when you prioritize your response to the situation. There is also an emotional undercurrent: you may be feeling things such as concern for Nilam, frustration at her mother, anger that no one has realized what the situation is, anxiety about the two-year-old. You will be acutely aware of the way in which your words and actions are affecting Nilam's wellbeing. For example, she says her mother is ill but you make the decision not to press her to name the illness; neither do you jump to any conclusions about the situation. You know that the decisions you make in this moment will have far-reaching effects. You may be holding conflicting ideas because you have not had time to check what the real situation is. You also have to manage this problem in real time, continuing with all other aspects of your role and aware of the safety and needs of the other children involved.

Your Reflective Timeline is in this moment, but is just one of many that will be occurring. Other professionals, such as the family doctor, social worker and occupational therapist, may be at different stages of reflecting about this family and their professional role. Nilam's burn may be the trigger for a new timeline for them, or a continuation of existing reflections.

Take a moment to move away from Nilam's story and think about an incident in your own work which has disrupted the normal running of your day: reflection in the moment happens in real time. A problem must be solved and you may have to think on your feet. Experience and your professional learning will already have taught you some of the skills you need. Your reflections are focused on making immediate decisions, but the more experienced and skilled you are the more likely you are to be thinking of the medium- and long-term consequences of your actions. Reflection at this time is fluid. It moves and jumps, accepting and rejecting decisions. Just like Nilam's teacher Mr Parker, you will be emotionally engaged. 'Emotional intelligence' is a phrase used to describe the way in which we relate to others, and use all of our senses to understand and inform our actions and behaviour (Higgs & Dulewicz, 2000).

Returning to Nilam, Mr Parker's thought process (much condensed) probably goes something like this:

Nilam is in pain and I'm concerned: why's she come to school like this? How did the mark get there? I've got twenty-five kids here ready for PE. I need help. Nilam's tired and upset. Alfie's got his head stuck in his tee-shirt. I need to take Nilam out of this situation but am responsible for this class. I don't want to send her away for help on her own. I need another adult here. Nilam is crying. Everyone is asking her questions. I need help fast. I'll send a child to get Mrs Fox here so I can concentrate on Nilam.

The teacher in this situation is using all of his *senses*. He knows from the noise in the room that the other children are becoming frustrated. They can *see* that Nilam is upset. They can smell that her clothes aren't washed.

Mr Parker has to cope with what is happening in the moment and with competing immediate needs. He doesn't over-reach himself by trying to deal with the class and Nilam

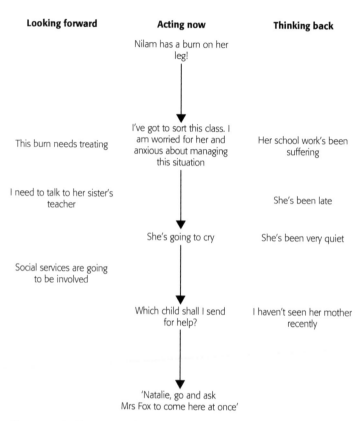

Looking forward	Acting now	Thinking back
	Nilam has a burn on her leg!	
This burn needs treating	I've got to sort this class. I am worried for her and anxious about managing this situation	Her school work's been suffering
I need to talk to her sister's teacher		She's been late
	She's going to cry	She's been very quiet
Social services are going to be involved		
	Which child shall I send for help?	I haven't seen her mother recently
	'Natalie, go and ask Mrs Fox to come here at once'	

Figure 3.3 Reflection in the moment

at the same time. A good reflective practitioner will always be thinking forwards and backwards to try to make sense of the situation. Figure 3.3 tries to capture the multiple thoughts that go alongside reflection in the moment.

Everything is going on at the same time. The teacher is supported by his professionalism and school safeguarding policy. By using reflection in the moment, the teacher is moving the situation forward safely.

Meanwhile . . . Sonja's mobile rings: a child has come to school with a suspicious burn on her leg; she is also talking about a younger child at home with a mother who is unable to get up.

As the duty social worker, this is where Sonja's timeline starts. In order to prioritize, she knows she needs more information. Nilam and her sister are in a safe situation until the end of school. The two-year-old could be at risk. Sonja knows nothing about the family; the situation could involve child abuse, domestic violence or the mother may be seriously ill. Sonja knows that there are likely to be other professionals already involved. Her professionalism has taught her that protecting a vulnerable child is the priority. She gets the address of Nilam's home and prepares to visit.

At this point we are going to leave Sonja's timeline, but you are welcome to develop it if you wish.

 EXERCISE

The next time that you are in a practice situation, try to capture a moment. Like a surfer riding waves, try to observe yourself in action. Ask yourself:

> What are the thoughts that are guiding your actions?
> Are there things that you already know that are guiding your actions?
> Are you thinking ahead as you act, to what you may need to do next, and to the consequences of your decisions?
> How do you feel? What impact does your emotional state have on your performance, actions and decisions?

▶▶ *Looking back*

Schön (1991) would call this reflection on action. This is where, after the event, you look back and re-visit your actions. Time has passed and your thoughts and feelings have changed. You will know some but not all of the consequences of your actions, and you will have had time to reflect on your own feelings. You may still have responsibility or you may have handed that over to other agencies. This is the point when you can be really critical in your analysis of your own role and professional practice.

Returning to our story: Mr Parker is now at home and

reflecting on the day. The central reflection is about Nilam and her wellbeing. He feels that the situation with Nilam was handled well and with the best possible outcome. But, analysing after the event, the teacher realizes that there were many signs that Nilam was struggling: missed homework, appearance, tiredness, all pointed to the fact that things weren't right at home. The value of fiction is that we can offer a possible explanation from Nilam's viewpoint:

Nilam's Story

Mum didn't get up this morning. It's six days now. Her pills isn't working and she can't tell the doctor in case she says Mum can't look after us. I made her tea and we had toast. It was the last slice. There's no bread in the freezer any more. I looked in the money tin and there isn't any more money. I changed Ali and put the washing in because it was smelly. I can put it on the radiators when I get home. But I don't know what I can make for tea. Don't put me in care. Mummy sometimes gets better then we'll go shopping and get lots of stuff for dinners. When she's good she can look after us. She said 'Look at your skirt, all crumpled, what will people think of me?' We were late, Ali was crying and I didn't have time to take it off. Can I go home now – she needs me?

And our story ends . . .

At the surgery, the nurse practitioner realizes that Nilam's mother has not picked up her repeat prescription. Knowing how important her medication is to her wellbeing, the nurse schedules a visit that afternoon. At the house, she finds Sonja (the social worker) and a neighbour. The neighbour has fed Ali and Mum. Sonja has arranged for emergency benefit to be paid, and the neighbour's husband has gone to the supermarket with a list made by Nilam's Mum.

Nilam has had the burn treated and an auntie will be staying the night. Some stories are over but others are just beginning.

Reflecting back

It's now time for you to reflect on this scenario. Everyone reflects differently and in different spaces. Some people go for a bath; some people walk; some people can reflect in lots of noise and other people need silence. There is no right way.

Start by thinking about the story; do not add to it and do not make any assumptions or fill in the gaps: reflection requires honesty and the gaps may be important. In the swampy ground of professional practice you rarely know all the facts, background or consequences of your actions, so this scenario is no different.

(1) Start by noting what you know. We have given you a thumbnail sketch of the incident and some of the professionals involved in Nilam's situation.

(2) Now be self-observant. What are *your* thoughts and feelings? If you told this story to someone else, how would you describe those involved? What would this reveal about your beliefs and attitudes?

(3) If this is a scenario where you, in your professional role, may have played a part, would you have made the same decisions? If your professional role is not in situations like this (you may, for example, work anywhere from an operating theatre to a prison), try to construct parallels where the unexpected happens and you have to think on your feet.

(4) Can you construct a scenario in which the actions and outcomes are different?

▶▶ *Looking again*

This is your opportunity to build on your reflective learning. It may be during supervision, as part of staff development, or on an education programme. It equates to Driscoll's 'So what?' stage (Driscoll, 2000). It may equally occur in private reflection. Perhaps a later incident jogs your memory and leaves you recollecting the incident, or you meet someone who was involved at a later date and learn more about the consequences.

The story has changed: it is now about you and your practice. This is when the lessons learnt form the pathway for your professional and emotional development. This is when you learn to do a job you do well better.

Looking again at Nilam's story from your professional viewpoint, what have you learned? Some immediate thoughts might be:

- keeping your head in a difficult situation can positively affect the outcome
- being worried or anxious can be normal aspects of an unexpected emergency situation
- professionals can rarely do everything themselves – we all need support
- keeping sight of the fundamentals – for example the well-being and safety of people we are responsible for – enables us to make decisions in uncertain situations

These reflections are no longer about Nilam. Looking again is about learning from any situation and how we apply that learning in the future. This process – what we learn about doing things well and doing things differently – is part of positive professional development. It will be important in later chapters, particularly where we look at coping with mistakes and whistle blowing in chapters 7 and 8.

▶▶*Moving on*

Often reflection is just about the incident, but effective reflective practice carries its learning with it. This is when reflective practice lies at the heart of your professionalism. You no longer do 'reflection': you are reflective. In simple terms, it is professional wisdom (Banks & Gallagher, 2009). It is the point at which you leave and move on. This is probably the least well understood and developed aspect of reflective practice, but crucial to the Reflective Timeline.

Returning to Nilam, time has passed and all the professional people involved in her family's crisis have moved on.

Mr Parker, the teacher, will still have Nilam in his class for the rest of the year. His relationship with her is altered by his new knowledge of her home situation. His reflection on action revealed a number of signs that, with the value of hindsight, may have alerted him to her problems earlier. He has reflected on his role as a teacher, and where the boundaries between 'just' teaching and the wider welfare and safety of the children in his class lie. He has had a positive experience of multi-agency working in which the social worker and health professionals have collaborated to keep Nilam and her family together and support them through a crisis.

All of this learning becomes part of the sort of professional he is. Like the cyclist in chapter 1, whose proficiency is enhanced by each journey, he moves on, embedding his learning into his professional development and everyday performance.

 EXERCISE

For the rest of this chapter, we want to take you through your own Reflective Timeline.

Recognizing in the moment

The reflection you are doing at this moment is reading this chapter. The story is about you and your learning.

How do you feel? Are you comfortable? Is this boring? Do you know this already?

In five minutes' time, your responses will be different. During those 300 seconds, you will have made decisions, thought more about Nilam's story in relation to your own practice, perhaps been interrupted and made judgements about how much more to read.

'In the moment' is sensory and immediate and quickly superseded by another moment.

We have used you reading this book because that is what you are doing now. The moment you look back on it or remember something from a previous chapter, your practice or your lectures, you are looking back and reflecting on your actions which are another part of the timeline.

1. Re-visiting the moment

How are you capturing this reflection? Professionals are often asked to keep a reflective journal, as part of their initial education and as a component of their continuing professional development. However, this takes time and effort and sometimes people 'cheat' by writing it up days or weeks later when they have to hand it in for assessment or supervision (Hobbs, 2007; Macfarlane & Gourlay, 2009); we discuss this in more detail in chapter 9. It is much better to capture it while it is fresh in your mind, so this is a chance to practise. As we will explore in chapter 6, your reflection can be written, but it can also take the form of a mind map, a picture, an audio recording – anything that will enable you to re-create the moment. It needs to be stored somewhere you can easily find it.

Have you chosen a method? Then let's continue.

2. If . . .

We all have incidents in our lives that make us think back over what we have done and use the 'if' word. We cannot change these moments, but we can use them to create a better understanding of ourselves and others.

Think of one of these moments. Try to recall it as accurately as possible. This will take longer than the moment itself. In chapter 4, we explore the legal status of documenting reflection, so, from this first moment, even in this private reflection, think about the words you use and where you store your thoughts.

Were you sitting or standing? Were other people involved? What had happened just before the moment? Was it raining? Were you in a hurry? How were you feeling? What were you wearing? If words were involved, what was said? What was the tone? What was said and what do you think was meant? When you have got as much detail as you possibly think you can, stop.

Take a break from it and come back in five minutes.

Welcome back!

Have you thought about the incident during those five minutes? Have you remembered other things? Now re-visit your first responses. Is there anything you want to add or change?

Where did that come from?

3. Analysis

Are there any themes or strands that jump out at you? For example: the way people communicated, the environment, your feelings, the professional standing of you and others and the effect on the people involved.

By doing this you are starting to analyse your reflection.

People can be frightened by the idea of analysis. But if you start by looking for themes that you can easily recognize, you can't go far wrong. Analysis is more than description, it is organizing and structuring that is geared to understanding (McMillan & Weyers, 2006).

Record the three themes that seem most important, and choose one of them to explore in more detail. For this theme, what do you know that helps you to understand it and to see how it applies to your 'If' moment?

For example, if your theme is about communication, you may be searching for theories about how people communicate, barriers to communication and so on. Does this theoretical application help you to break the moment down? Can you see things now that were 'hidden'? How does this feel? Are you vindicated in a decision you have made / uncomfortable because you can see ways in which you might have unintentionally contributed to a less than good outcome / puzzled by inconsistencies?

All of this is good. You are beginning to take analysis one step further and to be critical. This means that you are looking at the extent to which theory really explains or applies to prac- tice, searching for alternative explanations to the obvious and challenging assumptions – your own and others'. You might want to use a four-level structure (Smith, 2011) which asks you to explore the personal issues, interaction with others, theo- retical considerations and the political/social context.

How long you spend in this stage of the timeline will really depend on you. You may only have time to quickly explore one theme, but may equally now be really curious to explore this 'If' moment in much more detail and to look at other themes. You may want to search for other writing, research and theoretical explanations that help you to make sense of it.

 SEARCH AND EXPLORE

This may be a good point to search for information about one of your themes. Try putting a key word into your library search engine, or a global one on the internet. Where does this take you? What have you learned?

4. Leaving

But: there is a moment when you need to gather up your learning and leave. In our experience of working with health and social care professionals, when invited to recount an 'If' moment, people will often return to something deep in their past professional experience that has remained with them. The 'Janet's First Nights' reflection in chapter 1 is an example of this. You may also remember a wonderful cathartic moment that defines you and your professional image. However, such memories are often about unresolved emotions – a tragedy perhaps, or a missed opportunity.

In this case, the critical analysis above may help you to make sense of it, but it is easy to get stuck in the analysis, application of theory and critique stage, and never to move on.

So, for your 'If' moment, move on now: what have you learned?

This may be small things or fundamental self-revelations, it does not matter which – this is *your* moment, and, big or small, it's the learning that you take from it that is precious to you.

5. The future

What will you do differently, what has changed for you?

Again – this is very personal. Perhaps you will approach your practice with greater confidence in yourself and your abilities? Maybe you will recognize that you need supervision to overcome a particular worry, or maybe there is an area of learning that you now passionately and curiously want to follow up. Perhaps you have a new respect for a co-worker or the resilience of someone for whom you are responsible. All these are positive responses and should help to give you professional satisfaction.

6. And finally

What will you leave behind?

A snail leaves a trail, a part of itself that it no longer needs. This may be the moment in your reflection to leave something behind. This might be something emotional that maybe upsets or angers you and that you now realize is of no use to you and is getting in the way of your professional and personal development. Let it go!

It might be something you lacked confidence in doing. Your reflection has shown you that you can now do it well, so the old self can go. Whatever it is, leaving behind the things you no longer need to carry with you, which do not help you practically or emotionally, can be a very important and powerful part of being a reflective practitioner.

You have now completed the Reflective Timeline. We are

sure that none of the individual components of this will have been unfamiliar to you. However, putting them all together in a systematic way is important to developing reflective practice.

 EXERCISE

In demonstrating this timeline for reflection, we have tried to show that, whilst your reflections are unique to you, they will always run alongside other people, and that understanding the work of others is essential. If you would like to push yourself to look more critically at this:

1. Identify a report or other information in which an issue has been investigated. You may have access to 'serious case reviews', reports of complaints, or whistle-blowing records within the organization you work for. If not, you will not have to search for long on the internet to find a public report, or an activist website related to your professional area. Read it through in an open-minded non-judgemental frame of mind.
2. Now really analyse the issues raised. Look critically at the professions involved, the consequences of action (or inaction) and the ways in which policy or institutionalized practice affected the situation. Try Smith's four levels of critical reflection – personal, interaction with others, theory and political/social context – to help you to structure this (Smith, 2011).
3. How does your analysis square up with the WHO (2010) report? Can you place the situation you have looked at within this international context?

Summary

In this chapter, we have taken you through the Reflective Timeline. We have used this to illustrate how your professional role and its interaction with others affects the people you are responsible for, your colleagues and, importantly, yourself.

We hope that it has given you confidence to stop and think, to reflect, and to analyse your own and others' actions – and finally to move on when you are ready, taking your new-found learning with you.

In chapters 4, 5 and 6, we will guide you through writing for reflection and using other media. The work you have done in this chapter may form the basis of more detailed reflective recordings in these chapters.

Suggested reading for this chapter

Smith, E. (2011). Teaching critical reflection. *Teaching in Higher Education*, 16(2), 211–23.

Smith is one of several authors offering a 'critical' reflective framework, so a good one to read if you are ready to explore beyond your feelings and the immediate issues of your practice.

WHO (2010). *Framework for action on interprofessional education & collaborative practice*. Geneva: WHO.

This is an excellent report that puts the sorts of inter-professional issues we all face into a global perspective.

CHAPTER FOUR

Writing reflection for assessment: the individual voice

Chapter Summary

One of the most common ways for students to be asked to demonstrate their reflection is through writing. This can be in the form of a reflective journal, a piece of writing taking the point of view of a client or patient, or capturing dialogue. Sometimes you will be asked to write directly about yourself, at other times you will be writing about your relationships with other professionals and people you are responsible for. This chapter takes you, step by step, through the process of producing a piece of reflective writing. As you produce your reflection, it also asks you to think about how and what you write: about your own and others' practice, including the legal and ethical status of your text. Through studying this chapter and engaging in the exercises, you will be able to:

- plan for and produce a piece of individual reflective writing
- link your own reflection to analysis and reading
- explore the ethical and legal status of written reflection

Many university courses ask you to submit a reflective journal, or an essay which will be marked by your tutor. Our experience has shown us that students have a number of reactions to this.

Some are confident in writing an academic essay but have

no idea how to get started writing reflectively, so they either struggle to change style, or hope that by ignoring the reflective bits they will get by. Others think that reflective writing will be easy because they just have to tell a story; these students write a sloppy essay that lacks academic analysis and rigour. Both sets of students can be frustrated and angry when they do not get the marks they think they deserve. This chapter aims to help both types of writer.

If you generally do well at written assignments, then essay-writing advice may feel like revision, but if you work your way through the exercises, they will help you to develop a wider repertoire of writing styles. If you worry about writing and know that your marks could be better, the structure here will not just help you with reflective writing, but will have the added benefit of improving your ability in other written work.

Let's get started: most of you reading this book will have chosen your area of study because you are people who learn by being hands-on and doing. All of you have chosen a career path which involves working with and learning from others; writing implies introspection and solitude, so:

Why write?

Often when students are asked to write for reflective practice, they ask why they need to write things down when they can 'remember' what happened. The problem with 'remembering' is that memory is selective and often things we remember one day we have forgotten the next, and vice versa. How many times have you ended up in the supermarket desperately trying to remember the thing you came for, only to go home without it? Writing a list of what you need helps to solve this problem; it also has the added bonus of saving you time 'remembering' and needing to go back for something you have forgotten. Writing for reflection can help you save time by cutting out the need to re-visit something time and time again to collect all the facts.

Writing things down sets them in a particular time. If you are asked to reflect on your journey as a student at the end of the first year, you will have forgotten a lot of the feelings of newness, anticipation and anxiety you felt on the first day. In retrospect you may be able to remember that you were anxious, but not the list of things that contributed to the anxiety. You are now an expert on how long it will take to get to university and can spot the newbies who are walking round clutching maps trying to find impossibly named buildings. If reading this paragraph has made you remember that feeling, it has also shown you how quickly we forget things and feelings.

New technology has expanded on the way in which we can record things. We have a friend who regularly rings her home answer-phone to leave messages to herself about what she needs to have for work the next day. You, on the other hand, may hate to listen to the sound of yourself on the answer-phone, so use a note book. Others use their smart phones or computer note pad. In this chapter, all these ways of recording come under the banner of writing for reflection.

 TIME FOR REFLECTION

How do you work best? Think about the ways in which you record your thoughts and reflections. Make a point of having your preferred method to hand, and starting to note things as they occur to you.

There are times when you may be writing reflectively for assessment and are nervous about being honest because you perceive what you have to say as 'wrong' and think you will lose marks. One student Louise worked with was worried about writing a reflective essay about hand-washing because she had calculated that, if she carried out the recommended procedure, she would have been washing her hands for over three hours a day. When she reflected on the essay, she realized that the gap between recommended procedure and what could be realistically achieved in a busy hospital had an important point to make about why hygiene procedures get overlooked.

The tension between writing reflections that you think your tutor will be pleased with, and being truthful about yours and others' practice, can be difficult. Assessed reflections for health care students (Hargreaves, 2004) often follow one of three narrative lines. Firstly, the person reflecting narrates a situation in which they improve the outcome. Secondly, where something goes wrong and the reflection is about blame and guilt, the narrator shows what was done incorrectly and identifies the right course of action. Thirdly, through reflection the person narrating recognizes and changes some aspect of their own or others' practice. The argument goes that these are 'legitimate' reflections; they are likely to be viewed by others as demonstrating the right attitudes and understandings of the profession, and thus yield good marks. Reflections for assessments that do not follow these forms may be viewed as 'illegitimate' and, unless they are written very skilfully, are less likely to get the writer a good mark.

There is a small but growing area of literature challenging the value of assessment of reflection. See, for example, studies on reflective practice in teaching students, who write in their journals what they believe the tutor wants to read (Hobbs, 2007), the link between reflection and acting (Clegg, Tan & Saeidi, 2002), and the role that moving to online reflection may have in affective authenticity (Ross, 2011). The case against assessing reflection is discussed in more detail in chapter 9.

This chapter concentrates on writing with an *individual voice*; reflecting with others is different and will be discussed in chapter 5. Wherever possible, the exercises and illustrations are designed to be built into what you are already doing as part of your course, or your working life.

EXERCISE

Taking two of the reasons for reflecting we introduced in chapter 2 – 'recording thinking processes' and 'improving practice' – imagine you have been set an essay topic: *'Using reflective writing, assess an intervention you have made for a service user, and its outcome'*. Easy, you think: all I have to do is write about the one that makes me look best because that will get me the best mark.

Hold on!
Using the essay title above, this chapter will now walk you through the process of writing a reflective essay for assessment. We will explore:

►► the timeline for writing the essay
►► planning the essay: introduction and development
►► reading, research and references
►► re-writing and re-drafting
►► conclusion
►► moving on

►►The timeline for writing the essay

Illogical as it may seem, the easiest way to get a well-written essay in on time is to work backwards from the delivery date. For this illustration, we assume the essay length is 1,500 words; that the essay title has been given out at the end of the first week of the Spring Semester and it is due in on 1 April. This means that you have roughly twelve weeks in which to write your essay. Your first reaction has probably been 'Loads of time!', but look at the rest of the work which has to be handed in for marking. In all probability, you may have two or three pieces, all of which will have a similar deadline.

Find some sort of calendar which you can take in at a glance. Wall planners are excellent for this and there are all sorts of computer planners that you can print out. We suggest you create something that you can put up near the place you work and see easily (like table 4.1).

Table 4.1 The essay timeline

Week	Mon	Tue	Wed	Thu	Fri	Sat	Sun
1	Essay title given	Library & web search	Group work	Lectures	Library & web search	Working	Family time. Reading p.m.
2	Tutorial & placement prep.	Reading & thinking. Draft structure	Group work	Lectures	Library & web search	Working	Family time. Group work prep. p.m.
3	Tutorial & placement prep.	Hospital appointment	Group work	Lectures	Start first draft	Working	Family time. Work on draft
4	Placement	Placement	Placement	Placement	Placement	Working	Family time
5	Placement	Placement	Placement	Placement	Placement	Working	Family time
6	Placement feedback day	Review & complete draft 1	Group work	Lectures	Day off with friends	Working	Family time
7	Tutorial & exam prep.	Review draft 1	Group work	Lectures	Prep. for presentation	Working	Family time. Look at draft
8	Tutorial & exam prep.	Prep. for presentation	Group work presentation	Lectures	Library & web search	Working	Family time
9	Tutorial & exam prep.	Exam prep.	Day off pre-exams	Lectures	Exams today	Working	Family time
10	Reading & thinking	Re-drafting	Re-drafting	Lectures	Sort finances and shopping	Working	Family time
11	Tutorial & portfolio work	Portfolio work	Portfolio work	Lectures	Proofread and update	Working	Family time
12	Tutorial & portfolio work	Finish essay today	Hand in portfolio	Evaluation day	1 April hand in day!!	Working	Family time

Now mark off 1 April as the day on which you have to submit your essay. Next block off all the days on which you know you will not have any time to concentrate on your essay. These might be days you are on a work placement, your children's half-term, your birthday, days on which you are in paid work. Suddenly you will see that there is less time than you thought.

We are sure you have already experienced the stress of handing something in on time. You may have your own horror story of your computer giving up the ghost or your cat getting lost or the bus being late when you have to have the essay in by 9 a.m. The easiest way to avoid being in this situation is to aim to have the essay ready a couple of days before you need to hand it in. Mark this day on your calendar as the day you complete your final draft. Now have a look at the space you have for writing and find a date by which you can have your first draft complete. Moving back from that, look at when you need to start writing, sort your notes, finish reading, collect evidence and structure your essay.

▶▶ Planning the essay

It is easy to think that because you are writing from reflection all you have to say is what you did, why you did it and come to a conclusion, and therefore you don't need an essay plan. Many students think that planning an essay wastes time but, as with the shopping-list example at the beginning of this chapter, essay planning is one of the most effective things you can do to save time and effort when writing any essay. A good essay plan will mean that you stick to the subject. This means you will be able to concentrate your reading and necessary research on the topic in hand. Reading in depth will allow you to develop your ideas. It is the development and discussion of ideas that tutors are looking for when marking your essay.

By breaking your essay down into pieces with suggested word length, you will be able to see when you have too much material and when you do not have enough. It also enables you to keep an eye on the word count of the essay. For the essay we are using to illustrate this chapter, your word breakdown might be something like this:

Section	Word count
Introduction	100
Development	1,200
Conclusion	200
Total	1,500

▶▶ Introduction

Your introduction needs to tell the person marking the essay how you are going to answer the question. As people who have read a lot of essays, we will try and give you an idea of what is going on in the mind of your tutor when they mark your essay.

Here are three possible introductions: read them and decide for yourself which you find the most interesting one. Can you identify why you have chosen that one instead of the others?

(1) *The Oxford English Dictionary Online defines 'assess' as 'evaluate or estimate the nature, ability, or quality of'. In this essay I will evaluate the quality of an intervention I have made with a service user during my time at university. I will start by describing the nature of the intervention, the outcome and what I have learnt from it.*

(2) *Working in a hospital, I was shocked to discover that there were people I did not like. I thought my training had prepared me to be non-judgemental. Using Gibbs' cycle of reflective practice (Ghaye & Lillyman, 2006), I will explore how my response to a situation has led to a change in my professional practice.*

(3) *Reflective practice lies at the heart of my practice. It is something that everyone working in the field needs to know how to do. When you reflect, you think about what you have done, what you could have done and what you are going to do differently next time.*

The tutor who is marking your essay will have read thousands of similar introductions to essays. Example 2 goes to the heart of this book: the use of reflection and its role in the development of a confident and dynamic practitioner. The use of the word 'shocked' immediately tells the marker that the student has understood what non-judgemental practice should look like.

In Example 1 the student has felt the need to look up the word 'assess', which immediately makes the reader of the essay feel that the student is un-confident about what they are doing. The dictionary is referenced but the fact that it is 'Online' makes the tutor wonder whether the rest of the essay is going to have been downloaded and whether the sources are reliable.

The final example shows that the student knows what he is doing but has no referencing to back up the assertions made.

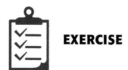 **EXERCISE**

Using one of the above examples, complete the rest of the introduction in such a way as to make the reader feel you know your subject and have relevant and interesting things to say about it. If you would like to use Gibbs' model, we have reproduced it as figure 4.1 to help.

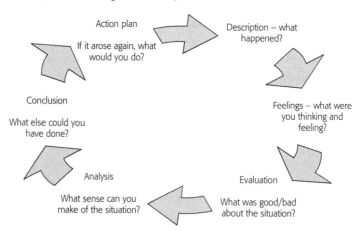

Figure 4.1 Gibbs' reflective cycle (Gibbs, 1988)

The truth of the matter about having your work marked is that, once you have lost the interest of whoever is marking the essay, it is difficult to get it back.

►► Development

1,200 words: that's almost a whole essay! The trick here is to break down the development of the essay into paragraphs. If you have ten paragraphs, that is only 120 words each. We're not suggesting that every paragraph should be exactly the same length, but it helps to have a rough idea. For the essay to read well and gain you vital marks, each paragraph needs to lead to the next one in a logical manner. Think of the times when people have told you stories and suddenly said 'Sorry, I missed a bit out.' In the academic world, there are no marks for bits missed out. An essay plan can help you make sure that this does not happen.

The paragraph above is exactly 120 words long. Once you start to break things down in this way, it's almost frightening how little space you have to tell your story.

Here we have broken down the development of the essay still further:

(1) What is the incident I have chosen and why have I chosen it?
(2) If I am using a reflective model, what is it?
(3) What was the setting for the intervention?
(4) Description of the intervention.
(5) What was my role during the intervention?
(6) What was my response?
(7) Could I have done something differently?
(8) What was the outcome?
(9) How did I feel at the time?
(10) How do I feel now?

You will see from this breakdown that, apart from (4), all the other items are questions that are looking for answers. It is the process of answering these questions that lets you explore your response to the situation in the light of your own knowledge and that of others. When you are writing reflectively, you are both the person asking the question and the one giving the answers. The hardest part of the process is resisting telling yourself what the answers are and allowing yourself to work towards them as part of the writing process.

Because reflective writing uses the first person 'I' and many of us are not terribly comfortable talking about ourselves and how we feel, let alone committing the process to writing, we can find ourselves embarrassed by our own presence in our narratives. Here are some tips for getting over that embarrassment:

- Never use 'i' instead of 'I'. You are training to be a professional; be proud of it.
- If your essay is reading 'I' at the beginning of every sentence, try changing the sentence structure around. *I was on the late shift* can become *The late shift started at 10 p.m.*
- This is your experience. Whether it was good or bad, you own it, and your experience of it is unique. That makes you the expert.

▶▶ Reading, research and references

Unlike a straightforward academic essay, the focus of your reading, research and references in a reflective essay will come from your own reflection and your expert knowledge of your field of practice.

 TIME FOR REFLECTION

Think about your own profession and a moment when you, or someone you observed, practised non-judgementally. What did it look like? How did you feel?

Let's take the second introduction from the exercise above as a starting point: the writer has not chosen 'non-judgemental practice' from a list of essay choices, or as a required topic. Rather, a reflection-in-action has led to a thoughtful and surprised response. This in turn is a springboard to thinking about non-judgemental practice and how it can be that, despite all the theoretical learning and strong personal desire to be a 'good' professional, you can still be stopped in your tracks because you find yourself disliking someone.

 SEARCH AND EXPLORE

Try searching on your university, or an open-access, search engine for 'non-judgemental practice'. Try other key words like 'discrimination' or 'prejudice' to widen your search. See if you can find two papers related to your profession, or an area of practice that you are interested in.

Look for papers that score highly with your key words, and then read the abstract to look for relevance and matches with the paper you are writing. When you have chosen some papers that you think might be relevant, read each through quickly, skimming for content and meaning, jotting down notes in whatever format you are using. Be ruthless! If you can see that the paper is not relevant, discard it and move on. Read again more carefully, write a short summary, mind map or bullet points. Highlight direct quotes that may be useful, being sure to include the full reference and page number.

Here is a worked example using two articles.

The first (Graham & Schiele, 2010) is a critical analysis of the ways in which 'race' as a focus of oppression and discrimination has changed over the past fifty years in the USA and the UK. The focus is social work education and practice, but the issues raised about anti-discriminatory or non-judgemental practice are universally applicable. The paper suggests that, because of changes in equality legislation, race is now seen as just one of many, equally important, aspects of a person, such as disability or sexual orientation. It goes on to argue that an unintended consequence is that the problem of racism has become diluted and thus is accorded less importance.

The second (Kiekkas, 2011) focuses on an intensive care unit, but again has wide applicability. It argues that, because of the intense, difficult working environment and human fallibility, the likelihood and significance of errors are high. The paper critiques literature around errors, and why they may go unreported. This includes lack of awareness and time, as well as fear of negative consequences, guilt and anger. A culture that fosters acceptance that errors happen is advocated. In doing so, the author cites research reports that link non-judgemental, positive error reporting with reduction of risk and improved practice.

Both of these articles, if used well, could be relevant in an assignment analysing non-judgemental or discriminatory practice. However, the way they are cited in reflective writing will be more personal, and include your own thoughts and feelings, as well as making links between theory and practice to explore, validate or question.

In order to illustrate this, we have written some paragraphs, using these citations in two different styles.

(1) For an academic essay critiquing non-judgemental practice, the papers could be used in the following way: *People may be treated less favourably for many reasons, including the colour of their skin, sexual orientation, disability or gender. The ways in which discrimination is defined, recognized and taught to professionals directly affect their behaviour. For example, Graham and Schiele (2010) argue that 'racism' is not considered to be as discriminatory in recent decades because it has been subsumed into a wider definition of 'difference' that hides its significance.*

Practitioners who have responsibility for the safety of vulnerable people are faced with pressure to avoid mistakes and cause no harm, in increasingly difficult and time-pressured environments. Kiekkas (2011) advocates a move to a 'shame free and blame free culture' (p. 4) in which errors are reported without fear in order to problem-solve effectively, and improve performance.

(2) However, using the same points in reflective writing, the paragraphs may look something like this:

I found myself returning to the moment I snapped at 'Stefan' over and over. Why had I been so abrupt in my manner? I saw his embarrassed and angry reaction and felt ashamed of upsetting him in this way. For a moment I had just seen him as an inconvenient problem at the end of a difficult day, not as a person. Graham and Schiele's (2010) critique of racial discrimination highlighted for me the ease with which individual differences can be lost in overall discourses about race, class and so on, and led me to re-examine the systematic way in which people can be marginalized by the very services that exist to support them.

At the end of the day, I returned home really tired and defeated. I was not happy with the way I had reacted to 'Stefan'. I desperately wanted to talk to someone about what had happened and to try to understand my reactions, so I talked to my supervisor. She was great. She let me talk about how I was feeling, and helped me to identify actions and reading that I can learn from. I am not surprised that this department has such a good reputation. The 'shame free and blame free culture' advocated by Kiekkas (2011, p. 4) for managing and reporting errors that is so evident in this place also affects the way that problems are talked about and solved for staff.

Reading, research and referencing, as you can see, are just as important in a reflective piece as in any other academic writing; it is the way they are explored, and incorporated into your text, that is different. In a reflective piece, personal experience and feelings are underpinned by the academic references.

 EXERCISE

Now it's your turn. Did you find some papers to read? Try summarizing them in your own language, avoiding 'cut and paste' shortcuts, so that you could explain the key points to someone else. Experiment with writing sentences and paragraphs that incorporate the reference into your reflective writing, so that your learning from reflection on action, and your theoretical analysis, are merged.

▶▶ Re-writing and re-drafting

Now you have written a draft, try to leave enough time to put it to one side and do something else for a few days, then read it through from beginning to end. How does it seem? Did you stick to your plan or drift off into another area? Do the paragraphs logically flow from each other? Go back to your essay title or instructions for the assignment. In this chapter, we gave the assignment: 'Using reflective writing, assess an intervention you have made for a service user, and its outcome', so we would expect:

- a reflective writing style – maybe following a model, if wanted or required
- a specific intervention with a service user
- a story of what you did and what happened
- assessment – a weighing-up of the value of what you did, using your reflective skills, literature and research

Many models of reflective practice encourage you to share your work with others. In her 'through the mirror' reflective writing, Bolton (2010) advocates asking a trusted friend to read and comment on your reflection. Many models, such as 'What? So what? Now what?' (Driscoll, 2000) and Johns' structured model (Johns, 2009) anticipate one-to-one supervision where the reflection is developed through a dialogue. If this is not possible for you, try reading aloud to yourself.

 SEARCH AND EXPLORE

There are several different software options that will read your essay to you. It can help you to improve your sentence construction and spelling, as well as making you reflect again about what you have written. Your university may offer this service, or try searching for 'read write software' and experiment with a free download that works for you.

Make alterations to refine and improve. Cross out sections that are not relevant or do not address the question. Edit sentences and paragraphs to make every word relevant and important to your narrative. How you do this will depend on your preferred style: you may like to print a copy and do hand-written alterations, or you may prefer to work on an electronic copy – whatever you do, number your drafts and keep them so you can go back to earlier versions if you need to.

▶▶ Conclusion

The conclusion is your opportunity to remind your reader of what you have written about and draw your writing to a close. It should not introduce any new points and, if you are using one, your reflective model may direct you – but if not, ask yourself:

- What are the main points that you have made that you want the reader to take away with them?
- Is there something in particular that you have learnt?
- Is there practice that has changed?
- Are there actions to be taken?

In our introduction, we put the spotlight on coping with disliking someone you have to work with, and assessing what this means in terms of non-judgemental practice. We then hinted at a change in practice as a result of this. The conclusion should mirror these points, drawing in this case on the action planning stage of Gibbs' cycle for support.

▶▶ Moving on

And finally, the reflective piece is written, you have checked all your references are included and correctly cited, presented it in the format required and saved it as 'final'. This may be the end of your writing, but is your reflection finished? Writing the reflection may have changed the way you think about this aspect of practice, it may have encouraged you to change something, or left you worried or upset.

Writing it down: the ethical and legal status of written reflection

Throughout your education as a professional, your development after you are qualified, and indeed everywhere in this book, we ask you to reflect. To think, write, doodle, draw, create, using any medium that helps you to explore your practice and stimulates your thoughts. In chapter 1, we argued that ethics was never far away from reflection, and that by thinking critically about practice, you add to your understanding of the complexities of decision making and the dilemmas and difficulties faced in everyday practice. In chapter 2, we said that reflective practice was, amongst other things, a way to *record your thoughts* and *move difficult situations forward*. In this chapter, we have walked you through all the stages of writing a successful reflective assignment.

We now want you to pause for a moment and consider the implications of your reflections from ethical and legal perspectives. To illustrate the issues involved, here are a few examples of practice that might lead to a reflection:

- You have had a difficult week. You are working with a colleague whom you do not particularly like. Their manner is patronizing and you feel that they know they are making you unhappy. You are not sure if you are being bullied, or if you are overreacting, but you know how their behaviour, and your reaction to it, is making you feel.
- You are working in a team where you become aware that some poor practice is known about and tolerated by others. Perhaps a colleague or colleagues are drinking alcohol during their working day, some petty pilfering of materials is happening, or corners are being cut.

• You are working alongside a group of colleagues in an emergency situation. You are not the leader – you may be a student or an observer – but you witness practice where, for example, a child is taken into care, a person is physically restrained or a life-threatening incident occurs. You may, or may not, judge that the right decisions have been made.

As you wind down and try to relax at the end of the day, firstly you look back and reflect (figure 4.2).

And now: you have settled down to complete an entry in your reflective journal. . .

So what do you write? And what is the ethical and legal status of your writing?

In chapter 1, we suggested that professional ethics should include the core virtues of care; respectfulness;

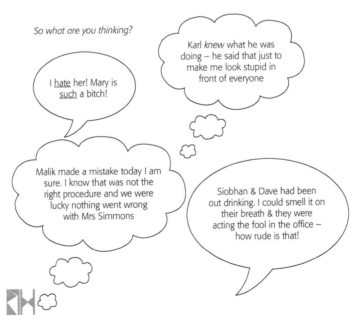

Figure 4.2 So what are you thinking?

trustworthiness; justice; courage; and integrity (Banks & Gallagher, 2009). They offer a guide to how we *ought* to behave as professionals. On the other hand, Dimond (2008) outlines the four arenas that govern how we *must* behave in order to work within the law (see also chapter 7 for a more detailed discussion). These are:

- criminal law
- civil law
- employment law
- professional codes of conduct

When you write something down it becomes more than just your personal reflections; because it is written down, it has a greater 'status' in terms of accountability. Things 'written down' include:

- a reflective journal entry
- a text on your mobile
- an essay
- a Twitter, blog or Facebook entry
- a formal report or professional account

Mary and Karl have upset you; these may be one-off incidents, but it may also be that they are bullying you and others, who may be more vulnerable than you and do not have a voice. Your initial reactions, thoughtfully recorded, may become the basis of a useful personal reflection, but may also lead to their professional practice (or your own) being challenged.

Malik, Siobhan and Dave's behaviour may trigger a professional investigation, threatening their employment and professional licence/registration. Siobhan and Dave at best are foolish, and at worst bring their profession into disrepute and may be a danger to others. You believe that Malik has made a mistake and Mrs Simmons was at risk. Can you simply record this and move on? What are your professional responsibilities?

TIME FOR REFLECTION

Think back to a moment when you have had similar thoughts of anger, disgust or dismay at a colleague's behaviour.

This may be your heartfelt reflection and you should not lose sight of the importance of your own emotional responses. We suggest that your sensory response is often the trigger for reflection, and capturing how you feel in the immediate moment is important. However, you must be mindful of the words you use. Box 4.1 includes some 'golden rules' for recording reflection:

Box 4.1 Golden rules for reflective writing

- Remember that *Anything* written down has legal status
- Always write only things that you know to be true: if you are unsure, say so (*I think she may have meant; I understood him to say that. . .*)
- If you want to express your reflection but cannot be 'truthful', write it as fiction, saying that this is what you have done – a poem or story may help you to reflect and move on
- Anonymize people and places unless you have a compelling reason not to – if necessary, change details to hide identity
- If you are required to name individuals, write with the expectation that the person will see what you have written; imagine them reading the actual words you have written. They may not like your reflection, but they should not be able to say that it's untrue or unprofessional
- Store your writing securely

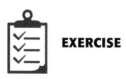 **EXERCISE**

If you want to improve your reflective writing a good way to do so is to read and critically analyse some published work.

1. Arber (2006) is an account from a Ph.D. thesis which is written in a powerful reflective style (and is openly accessible on-line). Read the work critically, looking at the language and structure used.
2. Now it's your turn – try using the styles you have read in this article, and others you have searched for in this chapter, in your own writing – don't be afraid to experiment!

Summary

In this chapter, we have offered you a detailed structure for writing a reflective assignment. We have used a conventional essay-planning style, illustrating how a reflective paper is similar to any written assignment in structure, but uses different language and writing conventions. We have also talked about the ethical, and possibly legal, significance of recording your reflections about live events and people.

Suggested reading for this chapter

Arber, A. (2006). Reflexivity: a challenge for the researcher as practitioner? *Journal of Research in Nursing*, 11(2), 147–57.

A good example of reflective writing for style.

Hargreaves, J. (2004). So how do you feel about that? Assessing reflective practice. *Nurse Education Today*, 24(3), 196–201.

This paper will come up again in chapter 9, but you may find it interesting to read now if you are thinking about the types of reflective accounts that you might write.

CHAPTER FIVE

Reflecting together: the collective voice

Chapter Summary

In practice, much reflection takes place in groups rather than individually. Group reflection brings with it another set of issues and debates: differences of perception, conflicting stories, competing truths and tensions between different disciplines. This chapter will explore how reflection can be shared between professionals without losing individual perspective and expertise. We will talk you through the process of organizing and running a reflective group yourself, and demonstrate that, used well, collective knowledge is stronger and better able to effect change than individual knowledge. Through studying this chapter and engaging in the exercises, you will be able to:

- understand the importance of shared reflective practice and inter-disciplinary working
- explore being part of a group whilst retaining your individuality
- listen to others without feeling threatened by their different perception of a situation

There is a lot of theory on groups and the way they operate. You will have experienced yourself the way you behave differently when you are alone, with your family, your friends or your professional colleagues.

TIME FOR REFLECTION

Stop for a moment and list the main groups that you are a member of. How many did you get to?

You may have included a group of people you work with, the whole student group for your course, or a sub-group; this may be friends whom you choose to associate with, but may also be a group designated by your course leader where you have no choice of membership. You probably have membership of some social groups too: you may be part of a family group, a member of a club or society. The size of a group can be very variable, from just three or four people to hundreds, or, in the case of a social network site, thousands of people may be collectively in touch with each other.

Your role within the group will also vary. In some, you may be the leader; in others, you may be an employee, connected by family or personal interests, or a volunteer. Some groups may have a defined purpose – to complete a work task or a piece of course work for assessment; others may be more open and less defined. In this chapter, we are interested in group *reflection*, so smaller groups where people are able to have a collective discussion are the focus.

 SEARCH AND EXPLORE

There is a huge amount of online information about groups. Try searching for 'group dynamics' to explore what 'sort' of group member you may be, and what an ideal group may consist of. But do not get sidetracked by this; we are more interested in group reflection, and how this can enhance your practice.

Why reflect in a group?

What is the weather like today? You may think it's a nuisance that it's snowing because you'll have to wear your coat and leave early. Your neighbour might be smiling because the slugs and snails will be killed by the cold. Children will be excited and drivers will be anxious.

If all of these people come together in a group reflection, their perceptions of the day and emotional responses will be very different. Group reflection on practice will contain similar differences of perception in which your beliefs and personal preferences will be challenged.

In earlier chapters, we have concentrated mostly on you as an individual. But in your practice as a student and your working life, you will usually be part of a professional group where people have different levels of qualification and responsibility. When you meet together to discuss your cases, professional differences and complex hierarchies will be involved. Reflecting on your own allows you to hold on to a particular opinion without being challenged. In a group, you have to accept somebody may disagree with you: by keeping an open mind, you may understand something differently and change your opinion. This openness is what all good practitioners aspire to.

Although few professionals work in complete isolation, most models of reflection are written as if they apply to an individual. It is also the case that a lot of reflective learning is taught in uniprofessional groups where 'professional boundaries and traditional delineated roles may be reinforced rather than reduced' (Karban & Smith, 2010, p. 176). Although reflecting on positive and negative situations is of equal importance, they argue that critical reflection in an inter-professional situation, which requires the exploration of wider social and political issues, will lead to professional decisions and professional differences being highlighted and challenged.

Fook and Gardner (2007) show how a four-stage model probing these wider social and political issues can form a valuable structure for bringing challenge and criticality into group reflection. Whatever the trigger for a group reflection, its purpose is to enable everyone to learn and move on. At its best, the outcome could be as significant as a change in the way services are delivered.

One of the reasons we are writing this book without a particular profession in mind is to encourage you to reflect personally and within groups, rather than just seeing issues from your own perspective. We have said that reflection has the capacity to embed good practice; record thinking processes; develop skills; improve practice; and, crucially, to move difficult situations forward. Group reflection can achieve all of these outcomes but can be destructive and unhelpful if it is not well managed.

In this chapter, we will include some pointers to literature that we think may be helpful but we are not offering a detailed critique of the literature on group work and group dynamics: this is well researched and published elsewhere. What we do want to do is to explore the space where personal reflection, reflective practice and being in a group overlap (see figure 5.1). The skills involved in personal reflection may not be the same as those needed for a group, and skilful group work is not necessarily reflective. By focusing on this area of overlap, we aim to help you to think about how to reflect in

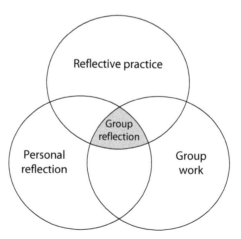

Figure 5.1 Group reflection

this particular 'space' and how you might facilitate reflection with others.

There are several things that are special about this space. You remain 'I', but you are also one of 'us'. You have a professional identity but also a team identity where the team members may all be of the same profession, but might all be different. Your personal and specialist views are just as important as when you reflect alone, but will need to be mediated through the group interaction. You will also have personal feelings and preferences about reflection.

 TIME FOR REFLECTION

Focus on an issue that you have been thinking about and look at the three rings of the diagram in figure 5.1. In which area would you feel most comfortable reflecting on this issue? Is the central group reflection the least or most acceptable to you? Why?

We all have different identities; the phrase 'Identity negotiation' (Swann, Johnson & Bosson, 2009, p. 82) describes a process that: 'transform[s] disconnected individuals into collaborators who have mutual obligations, common goals, and often, some degree of commitment to one another'. Negotiating who you are – your identity as an individual, professional and colleague within a group reflection – is an important part of your personal commitment to that group.

We have identified eight elements of a group that we believe will be significant in ensuring successful outcomes where the focus is reflection:

►► Getting together
►► People
►► Talking and listening
►► Being non-judgemental
►► Being 'in the room'

▶▶ Opening
▶▶ Contributing
▶▶ Outcomes

▶▶ Getting together

When you meet as a group, the first decision is where and when. This brings a structure to the meeting. The spontaneity you have when reflecting alone is lost. Arranging something at a time when everyone is available often leads to a least-worst scenario.

Where you meet is also a key factor. All space has connotations. We are most comfortable in our own space with our own things around us, but often you will be meeting in a space that you wouldn't choose, or somebody else's office. You may resent the time you spend going to an out-of-the-way place which has obviously been chosen for someone else's convenience. You may be used to reflecting in comfort but have instead to sit on children's chairs. You might like to move around when reflecting but now you are constrained.

There is also a time pressure. Very often, group reflection takes place at the end of the day. People are tired, worrying about getting home and already trying to plan the next day. You are not sure what is going to happen in the meeting, you may not even know exactly who is going to be there.

A further factor will be the reason for getting together. This may be a positive joint decision by a group of colleagues to reflect on their practice, or a management requirement where individuals feel they do not have a choice about joining in. Worse still, they may feel their 'performance' in the group is being assessed and judged by others. Where reflecting in groups is a 'requirement', spontaneity and willingness to engage may be lost (Platzer, Blake & Ashford, 2000).

EXERCISE

Identify a topic in your practice that would benefit from some group reflection. If you were going to organize this reflection, what factors would you take into account?

'Why?', 'What?', 'Where?', 'When?' and 'Who?' are not bad starting places. . .

Have a look at the group reflection checklist (table 5.1 on p. 104) to see whether you agree with our points.

▶▶ People

Who is in the room will influence what happens in the room.

Miller's reflection on her own role as a reflective group facilitator offers a powerful insight into reflective group dynamics (Miller, 2005). She talks about facilitating groups as being in a 'difficult and uncomfortable space' (p. 368) where the reactions of the people in the group and the outcomes cannot be easily predicted.

We all respond in different ways to things like superiority, experience, maturity and inter-professional dynamics. The group may be led by someone you trust and respect, by someone you do not feel that you can be honest with, or even by an external facilitator whom you have never met before. Equally, the members of the group may be a positive or negative influence on how you are feeling, and your willingness to engage.

 TIME FOR REFLECTION

Stop for a moment and think about how *you* come across in a group setting. How does it make you feel? Are you able to be open and comfortable, or do you feel defensive? What skills do you already have, and what might you need to develop?

Even if we don't like our manager or do not respect their professional knowledge, they are still our manager and probably exercise some sort of control over our job. Conversely, you might be the most senior member in the room with the ability to influence and control outcomes. The subject may be a sensitive one where it takes courage to raise difficult questions without being aggressive or defensive (see chapter 8).

Experience and maturity can often be confused. Someone who is younger may not have as much life experience and practice but might have the most up-to-date technical knowledge. We have all met 25-year-olds we would trust to behave well in all situations. We have all met 50-year-olds who get by on a wing and a prayer because it has worked for them in the past. Age should not be relevant to the quality of what a person can contribute to the group.

Inter-disciplinary dynamics will always be significant. Unfortunately, society sees certain roles and professions as being of more value than others. In practice, these roles rely on a significant contribution from other professionals. The surgeon may lead an operation but relies on a team to ensure the operation works smoothly. Once out of the operating theatre, another team takes over to ensure recovery, rehabilitation and discharge. For some patients, going home may lead to the involvement of social workers, occupational therapists, community nurses and others. Each of these professionals has a part to play in recovery. All their contributions are significant and should be valued as such.

You have chosen a particular profession because of your interest in it. Very quickly you will have picked up from your tutors and those you are working with the core values and focus of your profession. For example, a social worker will rate anti-discriminatory practice very highly, a physiotherapist works from close observation of the skeleton as well as what the patient tells them, a nurse is most likely to be concerned with caring for a person's immediate mental or physical needs, a dentist can probably assess a patient's diet from the state of their teeth.

▶▶Talking and listening

While inter-agency working is seen as an ideal, often in practice people are reluctant to share across boundaries. Sometimes they feel that, by sharing it, they are 'giving away' their expertise. But in many cases, it is only by accurate sharing and assessing of information that a whole picture can be built up. Each person holds a different piece of the jigsaw.

Each profession has its own distinctive language. Often this consists of shortcuts and acronyms which have immediate relevance to your subject area. While acronyms can be a useful shortcut when used between two professionals from the same subject area, they can also form a barrier for others.

 TIME FOR REFLECTION

Think back to when you first started to study your subject. Did you find yourself excluded and distanced by the way in which people were using language you didn't understand? Now your understanding of that language defines you as one of 'us'. But think back again to that feeling of exclusion: that is how other people feel when we use phrases and words that they do not understand in a group situation.

Sometimes in group reflections the participants are invited to stop and ask for clarity if they do not understand something. In practice this rarely happens: people are reluctant to say that they don't understand things and often think that asking for an explanation will hold up the meeting or expose their ignorance.

What is not said is often as important as what is said. Listening is not just about understanding words, but about interpreting silences. Reluctance to speak may be because someone is afraid, feels they won't be listened to, thinks the reflection a waste of time or is reluctant to share what they know with others.

Understanding these interpersonal dynamics is important for effective communication in reflective groups.

EXERCISE

Talking and listening in pairs:

Working with a colleague (if possible from a different discipline), ask them to talk to you for two minutes about a work event. Let them talk; do not interrupt or ask questions. When the two minutes are up, reverse the process and talk for two minutes yourself.

Now tell the other person what they told you. They must not interrupt. Now it is their turn to repeat what you told them.

Was this easy or difficult? Did you want to keep asking for extra information or were they getting their point across in a clear and concise manner? How did you do?

If you disagreed with them, how easy was it to get their points across? Were you able to be a dispassionate reporter?

Now you can have a reflective conversation about the process and what you learned.

▶▶ Being non-judgemental

You will have learnt during your studies the importance of being non-judgemental and not making un-justified assumptions. In practice this is very hard. We all make assumptions about people the moment we see them. Their hair, what they wear, how they move, their height, their weight – this is our fight-or-flight response coming into play. This happens in group reflective practice too, however hard we try not to judge from what we see. Walking into someone's office and seeing a picture of Elvis makes you think one thing about them; a picture of Beyonce would provoke a different response. Assumptions about their choice in music will interact with your own preferences, to influence how you think about them.

Body language and tone of voice, as much as what is and is not said, influence our judgements. The type of language used as well as things like tone or loudness; non-verbal cues such as eye contact, touch and closeness can all convey meanings that reinforce or contradict the words used. Also, if notes are being taken, the choice of what is recorded will be significant

(Thompson, 2009). We notice someone shifting awkwardly in their seat, the person who will not make eye contact with the group, the endless shuffling of notes by another. As non-verbal, as much as verbal, communication is cultural, we need to know that gestures and expressions may be misinterpreted unless we are culturally aware (Hook, Franks & Bauer, 2011).

You can see that taking a moment to think about how others are coming across to you is important, but so is your own behaviour: do you come across as making eye contact or are you staring? Is it obvious that your mind is elsewhere because you are playing with your phone? Are you nodding agreement but sitting with your arms tightly folded?

►► Being 'in the room'

Group reflection will usually focus on an area where people are emotionally engaged – this may be a critical incident or serious case review. The people involved are often nervous and frightened of what the outcome of the reflection will be. Therefore, in common with all group work, establishing ground rules and boundaries is important before the reflection starts (Bolton, 2010; Fook & Gardner, 2007). We have already covered a number of aspects of this: choosing where and when to meet, and being non-judgemental and prepared to listen openly to others are important starting points. Recording the session, agreeing length, and facilitation are further factors to take into account.

Deciding what sort of record will be kept will be part of establishing ground rules. Flip charts are an excellent way of doing this because everyone in the group can see them and they are easy to refer to. Other groups appoint a minute-taker. Taking minutes often means the person keeping them is so busy writing things down that they don't have a chance to contribute to the discussion. To avoid this situation, it is often a good idea to revolve the role of minute-taker. In formal situations, the meeting might be recorded to provide a lasting record.

Mr Mendosa did not seem to be moving when I came into the room. I was very concerned about him. He was slumped sideways in his chair and his breathing was laboured. When I called Anna she seemed rattled and immediately started speaking loudly to Mr Mendosa and getting him to sit up straight. He was very stiff and uncomfortable, and struggled to straighten himself up.

The person narrating could be from just about any profession, and the setting could be his home (Anna might be a family member), a care home, institution, police station or acute hospital setting. Put yourself in the shoes of 'I' in this story: you are in a group reflection focusing on Mr Mendosa's case.

If the reflection is occurring in a work setting, where the participants have a role in Mr Mendosa's care, there may be detailed factual discussions about his situation, care and outcomes of interventions. Here the ground rules may include confidentiality within the team, and a no-blame attitude. Formal notes may be taken, particularly in order to record decisions and actions.

If, however, you are part of a study group and have offered this incident to the other participants for discussion, the ground rules may still involve confidentiality and a non-judgemental approach, but your professionalism will mean that you do not reveal Mr Mendosa's identity or that of other people involved. Any notes taken will be about thoughts and feelings, and actions that group members may want to leave with, rather than details of the case.

In either situation, real consideration needs to be given to the discussion and the record of the reflection. This, like all other recordings of reflection, may be significant and you may want to refer back to the 'golden rules' of reflective writing suggested at the end of chapter 4, in box 4.1.

Deciding how long the reflective group is going to meet for is also important. Sometimes time constraints are an issue and it is important to resolve these at the beginning of the reflection. Having a time constraint can be very useful. When collaborating on this book, knowing we had limited time to write together meant that the time we had was focused and targeted. Time may relate to the length of a single session, or a number of sessions over time. Miller (2005) and Bolton (2010) both write with the expectation and experience as facilitators of working with a group over a period of several sessions. Fook and Gardner (2007) specifically advocate at least three meetings.

If someone has a pressing reason to leave early, it might be sensible to make sure they get a chance to make their contribution as soon as possible, rather than everyone having to meet again to hear what they have to say. However, it may also be agreed that the group finishes when people have to leave, so that they are not excluded from the discussion, or that everyone, as part of their responsibility to the group, commits to the time agreed.

The decision to have a chair or employ an external facilitator will also be a significant factor in the conduct of the reflection. It may be that a senior person has called the meeting and is automatically expected to chair, creating, or reinforcing, a power dynamic. By contrast, external facilitation may be either welcomed or a focus of aggression, as Miller (2005) has shown. If the chair is a volunteer, or elected from the body of the meeting, they need to have the skills to lead the group, and the support of others for this to be effective. Bolton suggests that facilitation, rather than leadership, is needed, her ideal is to create circumstances in which people lead themselves, and she suggests six attributes that are needed: 'responsibility, trust, self respect, generosity, positive regard and valuing diversity' (Bolton, 2010, p. 161).

▶▶ Opening

Having established the ground rules, the language used to introduce the subject of the reflection should be as neutral as possible. Consider the following introduction:

We've all been dragged out of bed early to try and sort out what went wrong with poor Mr Mendosa.

This is not neutral language. There is an implication that we are reluctant to be at the meeting: 'dragged'.

'Try and sort out what went wrong' implies that whatever went wrong was as the result of a mess of some sort.

'Poor Mr Mendosa' makes a value judgement about the client in question.

A more open way of starting this discussion might be something like: *The reason we are all here is to reflect on Mr Mendosa's case.*

The opening is also the opportunity to decide whether a particular model or approach is going to be used. A range of models have been introduced in chapter 2 for you to choose from and – particularly if this is a difficult situation, or you are unused to group reflection – the use of a model may help to manage the discussion.

▶▶ Contributing

You may hope that in a professional group reflection, everyone present has come prepared and ready to contribute. At best, there is an 'interpersonal glue' that can bind people together (Swann et al., 2009). However, the literature researching group dynamics explores the difficulties with this assumption.

Group dynamics can have a negative effect on performance of the group (Lepine & Van-Dyne, 2001). These authors suggest that the group 'moderates' poor performers through group-work, training, compensating or allowing for differences, rejection, or trying to motivate them to behave differently. You will probably all have tried at least one of these actions with a group you are a member of, but work-based groups are particularly difficult. Power dynamics and job hierarchies come into play; you will most probably have no control over who is in your group, so rejecting a disruptive member may not be an option. In addition, the imperative to maintain the professional service or role you perform may mean that tackling difficult group members is low on the list of priorities.

'Bad apple team members' (Felps, Mitchell & Byington, 2006) are people who don't do their share of the work, who are negative, bring the spirit of the group down or behave in an inappropriate way. Examples include silly jokes, making fun, inappropriate remarks and pranks. Similarly to Lepine and Van-Dyne (2001), they say that coping strategies include trying to motivate the person, or alternatively rejecting them – either literally if possible, or through minimizing interaction and contact where not possible. They suggest these strategies have the potential to be constructive but that, where the person has power or their negative effect is particularly strong, then the group reaction is angry and defensive, which can be very destructive for the group.

 TIME FOR REFLECTION

What sort of group member are you? Take a moment to think honestly about the way your contribution affects the groups you are a member of.

Many of the things we have already discussed, such as ground rules and clear purpose, will help to maximize positive contributions, but a further issue is that some people try to dominate groups by talking at great length. These people don't like being interrupted and it can be difficult to challenge what they are saying. Possible solutions to this might be:

- pointing out that other people want to contribute
- making sure they stick to agreed ground rules – for example, talking about practicalities not personalities.

Other people interrupt and talk over contributions. In this case it is permissible to say that their turn to speak will come or that they have already been listened to by the group. There will always be people who struggle to talk in a group. They are shy, they think their English isn't good enough or they feel intimidated by others in the room.

We have all been in meetings where this has happened! One of the ways this can be overcome is by giving people the same amount of space to talk and have their views listened to.

Rather than giving everybody five minutes to speak, a simpler and more effective way is to give everyone six tokens. (In her work Louise uses a tin of buttons, but you could use sweets, matchsticks, even torn-up pieces of paper.) Every time someone makes an intervention, they use up one of their tokens. People who talk a lot use up their tokens very quickly: this leaves the floor open for those who are reluctant to speak. By the time everyone has used their tokens, the reflection is usually in full flow and people have understood the importance of listening to others, but if this has not happened in your group you can easily re-allocate the tokens.

Outcomes

Reaching an outcome from the reflection that is acceptable to the group is important: there would be little point in spending time doing it if not. However, forcing, or pre-judging, the desirable outcome is equally pointless. Miller (2005), Fook and Gardner (2007) and Bolton (2010) are all in a position to talk about group reflection as an exercise supported by skilled facilitation over a period of several meetings. This may not be possible for you. You may have just one group reflection where you need to try to explore and reach some resolution to a problem. Be realistic!

Like Aladdin, you may have let a genie out of the bottle and raised many issues that cannot easily be resolved. People may have been emotional, and areas may have been raised that cannot be concluded within the time available. Bolton (2010) reminds us that everyone present will have made a contribution but, however important the group may have been, the learning is for each individual: what this is, and what it contributes is unpredictable, may be unexpected and may not be shared with the group.

Ensuring time is left at the end of a group reflection to sum up, debrief and agree actions will help to manage these issues. Returning to Mr Mendosa . . .

We recognize that we could have communicated better about Mr Mendosa's care and he should not have been put at risk. We are re-assessing our processes for passing information between the relevant services. This is a collective responsibility and we are meeting next week to begin implementation.

Mr Mendosa was put in an unfortunate situation, but as a result of group reflection changes will now take place. People are not blaming each other and individuals have had a chance to say how things could be made better. This may well be something they have felt powerless to say as an individual, or something they recognized but had not been able to see a solution for. As a result of what has been said in the room, everyone is now able to move on.

You may be thinking that group reflection is going to be difficult, fraught with interpersonal tensions and risk – however, the potential for valuable change is well worth striving for, and the checklist at the end of this chapter should help you to prepare well. There are many published examples of excellent group reflection, for example research around group reflection to improve hospital food preparation (Glina, Cardoso, Isosaki & Rocha, 2011).

 EXERCISE

A group does not happen by chance, it is created. If you are interested in critically analysing group reflection:

1. Take Miller's (2005) article and read it through. It's a good read – an eloquent narration from a skilled facilitator. Ask yourself what it tells you about her and her role. Think about how the participants in her groups might feel about the emotionally charged situations she narrates. Put yourself in their shoes, and hers.
2. Use Fook and Gardner's (2007) four stages to structure a group reflection that you lead. This model will encourage you to probe deeply beneath and beyond the immediate event, to challenge your own and others' conceptions and the infrastructure of the service you are engaged with. Remember this will need several hours with a committed group.

Summary

In this chapter we have focused on reflection in groups. To summarize, we have created a group reflection checklist (table 5.1), which we hope will help you to plan for, and positively contribute to, groups of your own.

Table 5.1 Group reflection checklist	
Why & what?	First things first: why are you meeting? Can you in one succinct sentence write down the reason for meeting so that it will be clear to others? If you are in a group reflection and you are not clear about the purpose, don't be afraid to ask!
Who am I?	What role are you going to play in the meeting? Are you the leader? What responsibility do you have to yourself, others in the room, the service . . .? Try to be really clear about this. If you enter the meeting knowing that you have strong judgements about the focus, or people in the room, or have intentions to be disruptive, think carefully about why you are doing this and what you want to achieve.
Where & when?	If you can choose the venue and time think about space, freedom from interruption, comfort, accessibility, convenience for all.
Time	How long do you have? Will you have one short meeting, or is there a commitment to several sessions over time? How long you have will be important in framing your 'why?' – one short group reflection is not going to change the culture of an organization, but if it's all you have, it might help a team to reflect on and resolve a difficult incident, leaving them stronger and more united.

Table 5.1 (continued)

Leadership	How is the reflection going to be facilitated? One or more of the group needs to take responsibility for opening and closing the session, keeping time and, if agreed, keeping a record. If there is no obvious leader, the group needs to agree these roles. If there is a person who is more senior than others, they need either to take the lead, or to be very clear about supporting whoever is facilitating.
Ground rules	Time spent agreeing the ground rules will pay off as the group progresses. If nothing else is written down, these should be. If the group meet regularly, either the rules need pinning up in the room, or everyone should have a copy.
Crowd control	A clear purpose, timeframe, ground rules and cue questions / model will help to manage the discussion. Both facilitator and group members should be prepared to 'police' this – e.g. if the ground rules agreed are that no one speaks aggressively, or prevents someone from speaking, all the group have to stand up for others if this happens.
Time-keeping	Keep an eye on time, and make sure to leave enough space to conclude, agree actions and debrief.
Personal conduct	Finally, the attributes of virtue ethics, introduced in chapter 1, are a good set of personal goals to aim for: care – for and about others in the room respectfulness – for others as well as self trustworthiness – to trust and be trusted justice – to be fair in what you say and giving others time to speak courage – to ask difficult questions and accept challenge integrity – to be true to oneself and others (Banks & Gallagher, 2009)

Suggested reading for this chapter

Bolton, G. (2010). *Reflective Practice: Writing and Professional Development* (3rd edn). London: Sage Publications.

Chapter 9 of this book specifically deals with facilitating group reflection – it's a good read, and offers practical help.

Fook, J. & Gardner, F. (2007). *Practising Critical Reflection: A Resource Handbook*. Maidenhead: Open University Press.

This whole book is devoted to developing a model of critical reflection that can be used to structure a group. It asks you to go beyond the immediate situation to critique social assumptions and political/cultural implications. It is challenging and may offer a useful structure if you are trying to get beyond the 'I think, I feel' stage and on to something that is more deeply embedded in the discourses of your profession.

Miller, S. (2005). What it's like being the 'holder of the space': a narrative on working with reflective practice in groups. *Reflective Practice*, 6(3), 367–77.

This is an interesting read – useful as an example of reflective writing, and insightful with regard to facilitating a group – in terms of the role you might have to take yourself, but also of understanding how it might feel to be an external facilitator.

CHAPTER SIX

Expressing reflection in other ways

Chapter Summary

In the previous chapters we have concentrated on written reflection; this chapter looks at other forms of reflection that don't involve writing, and how they can be embedded in good practice. Non-written individual and group reflections are suggested as well as the use of digital media. We also give you some ideas for ways of developing practical reflections for yourself and others. Though some of the ideas may at first feel uncomfortable, by engaging with this chapter, you will be able to:

- reflect without using the written medium
- develop skills to involve others in reflection
- discover that reflection can take different practical forms

There is so much more potential in reflective practice than just using the written form to explore and record reflection and we aim to inspire you to experiment with some of this diversity in this chapter. However, before looking at the ways in which all of our senses can be used and suggesting some practical exercises, we want specifically to review digital reflection.

Reflecting digitally

A significant development in reflective practice has been the availability and use of digital media. We have suggested in other chapters occasions when you might be using electronic, rather than paper-based, ways of recording your reflections. This might be taking a photograph on your mobile phone, using a device to record your thoughts or simply calling your own phone at home to capture a reflective thought. You may also find yourself expected to keep an electronic portfolio, write your reflective journal as a blog, or join an on-line reflective conversation. Looking at the literature, it's clear that in some cases digital delivery is just a different way of doing the same thing; calling a reflective learning journal a 'blog' does not in some magical way make it any more or less significant than its paper-based cousin.

However, the development of digital portfolios offers huge potential for reflecting and demonstrating reflection in different ways – for example, adding artefacts such as video clips and mixed media (Montgomery, 2003); they also offer the opportunity for instantly sharing with others on-line, so more immediate discussion, supervision and feedback can be obtained. A further factor regarding internet use is that it offers an opportunity for university-based tutors to keep in touch with students once they are in placements. This raises the opportunity for continued supervision of reflection when students may feel isolated from their university tutors and confronting professionally challenging situations for the first time (Rhine & Bryant, 2007). In Rhine and Bryant's research with trainee lecturers, digital media are used to video their classroom delivery and then shared on-line to facilitate tutor and peer discussion. In a related project, medical students were required to log exchanges with patients and record learning points on mobile devices (Thomas & Goldberg, 2007). The immediacy of the recording made keeping a record in very busy clinical practice possible in a way that retrospective journals could not have done. In different ways, the two projects allowed for reflection because of the technology.

Use of the internet allows for global communication; for example, in Gardner et al. (2012), dentists in six countries use a web platform to facilitate collaboration and reflection. Their aim is to use reflection in dental education as a medium for thinking about practice and being empathetic with patients rather than seeking 'set answers to set problems' (p. 208); the authors had been running the scheme for five years at the point of publication. They argue that the project creates a community of practice between the students where they develop 'global citizenship'. They collaborate on an assessment through which they learn to communicate in a professional and intelligent way but with kindness and warmth. A measure of its success is that students develop videos and other creative artefacts beyond the brief of the project.

Not all digital developments are on-line: digital stories are usually short accounts of a person's life, or aspects of their experience, that are shared to facilitate understanding and reflection (Sandars & Murray, 2011). Oral and visual artefacts can be used with students to create a digital story about aspects of practice, which can be part of a learning process and may be submitted for assessment.

 SEARCH AND EXPLORE

There are many digital stories deposited on-line. Search for 'digital stories' or 'patient voices' and you will find a wealth of examples. They are worth looking at in their own right, but also are particularly useful as triggers for personal or group reflection and as examples of a non-written way of conveying an experience or message.

So, you can see that digital resources can be used to express reflection in non-written forms, facilitate communication where face-to-face contact is not possible and widen horizons by allowing for global communities of students to form. They open a whole new aspect to portfolios that can use different media and be shared selectively with others. Whilst the literature is generally positive, the same challenges exist here as with any medium – for example, student engagement and the difficulties of assessment – which are discussed in more detail in chapter 9.

A rare note of caution that may be particular to digital reflection concerns the ways in which on-line reflection 'amplifies' the surveillance elements of reflective practice (Ross, 2011). Ross' research explores the experiences of people reflecting in digital forms and has led her to assert that it produces a very different form of reflection. She argues that the potential for constant monitoring by others and the openness of the digital world affect the ways in which people portray themselves. She uses the analogy of wearing many different masks and suggests that constant contact via the internet, which may be supportive and positive, can also be oppressive and controlling. In chapter 4, we discussed the ethical and legal status of written reflection; the golden rules listed later are perhaps even more relevant for digital reflection. Whilst you can destroy or restrict access to paper-based reflections, it may be beyond your control to retrieve and erase something you have recorded electronically, such as a blog or a tweet.

Professionals have different ways of reflecting

Most professionals use reflection in some way. For example, it would be impossible to become an architect without looking at buildings and thinking about them. When we look at a building, we quickly make a decision about what it is – for example, a hospital looks different from a house and a school looks different from a shopping centre. Old houses are built of different materials and to different specifications from new ones. But each building has a narrative in much the same way as a story has a narrative. Before it can be designed and built, the architect must think about its use, its construction and materials.

The performing arts also use reflection. This time it is in the form of rehearsals. Musicians work together to make sure they are in tune and in time with each other. Dancers go back over moves until they have a fluency of performance. Much of the reflection that these practitioners use is done through their bodies. Actors will often say in rehearsal that something does not 'feel right'. They go back and change what they have done – perhaps moving to a different part of the stage or picking up a prop.

Aristotle defined the five senses as being sight, sound, touch, taste and smell. We store reflection, in the form of memory, through these senses. In their most basic form, they are part of our fight-or-flight response (Jenkins & Tortora, 2013). However, with experience, we add to them emotionally and intellectually.

 SEARCH AND EXPLORE

If you search for Aristotle and the five senses, you will find a lot of information on-line. Since Aristotle's time, other senses have been attributed to humans. One you will certainly be aware of is time – have a look and see what the others are. Do you think there is anything missing?

Through our senses, we notice very small changes to familiar things:

- the choice of a slightly different colour on a letter-head, or when someone's hair goes a couple of shades blonder
- we remember the taste of another cup of coffee and whether it was better or worse than the one we are drinking now
- we hear a snatch of our favourite song and it gives us a feeling of wellbeing and happiness
- our hands reach out to stroke a piece of velvet that reminds us of our favourite toy
- the smell of fresh baked bread makes us want a slice

TIME FOR REFLECTION

Think about your favourite toy when you were a child. Which of the five senses does it bring to mind most strongly? Why?

The German philosopher Immanuel Kant whom we mentioned in chapter 1 said that there were two sources of understanding. These he described as sensibility – meaning time and space – and understanding – meaning things we have not learnt from experience but are able to interpret to make sense of our experiences. He believed that the power to reflect upon experience helped people to develop a greater knowledge of themselves and the world around them (Pirie, 2009).

This chapter now devotes itself to suggestions for reflections that can be done without writing. They are offered to you to do in your own time or to use as part of a group reflection. Hopefully, we will have included something in this chapter that you will be prepared to try out as part of your practice and which will enrich your understanding. These are all exercises we have done with students and professionals, which have helped them to develop different ways of reflecting on their practice.

 EXERCISE   **TIME FOR REFLECTION**

Think back to an incident which puzzled you. Gather the main things that you remember in your thoughts. Jot them down or draw a diagram if that helps. You are now going to try to reflect on it in a much more physical and sensory way than by writing.

Try to remember the smell. A smell of burning might tell you that someone with memory problems has forgotten to turn off their oven.

Did you hear anything differently? Perhaps a client's voice was quieter or louder than usual.

What did the things around you feel like? Did they feel dirty and gritty or perhaps you remember your knuckles as you clutched your bag or clipboard.

Taste is more difficult in these situations. Was the milk on the turn or the biscuit you were offered stale?

Light moves at 299,792,458 m/s. In practice, this means we often see something and make a judgement before we have had time to engage with it in any other way. *Was something different as you walked towards the bed? Did a client appear more carelessly dressed than before? Was the person in front of you nervous?*

The experiences above are mostly negative, but don't ignore the positive. Perhaps the person you were with was more talkative than usual. They may not have said 'I'm feeling better' but for someone who has been depressed and unhappy a sentence like 'Aren't the leaves beautiful today?' is a real step forward.

We have learnt as teachers that sometimes our students seem to grow in front of our eyes as they become more confident and gain better marks. Of course, they have not grown physically, but their progress and pleasure is reflected in their whole demeanour. Has this happened to you or anyone you know?

Adding these elements of sensory reflection together, have you been able to add to your understanding of what was going on?

Picture it

Thanks to new technologies we are living in a very visual world. We spend much of our time being bombarded with information which comes to us in a very visual way.

Our knowledge enables us to decode images and what they are conveying to us. Globalization means that producers and advertisers are trying to reach the biggest possible market. Campaigns that work on images that can be understood whatever the language spoken mean a greater reach for the product.

Many of you as students will have been asked to develop posters to convey information. This is a pictorial way of reaching as many people as possible. The KAWA reflective model uses a cross-sectional picture of a river in which you are encouraged to build up your personal reflection, using the depth and breadth of the river and obstacles such as rocks to represent your personal reflection. By using a picture and the familiar structure of a river, it transcends language and culture.

You will be familiar with pie charts but did you know they were popularized by Florence Nightingale who wanted a visual and shocking way to show the British army what was causing soldiers to die? Showing statistics in such a diagrammatical way made them easier to understand than a list of numbers and helped her to win supporters to her cause.

 SEARCH AND EXPLORE

Just type 'Florence Nightingale' and 'pie charts' into any search engine and you will be able to see images she created. There are many biographies of her work. Bostridge (2008) is a recent and comprehensive account.

Schools, universities, sports clubs, businesses and others all try to brand themselves by using logos. These are images which represent the brand. The Buckingham Report (DCSF, 2009) is an assessment of the impact of the commercial world on children's wellbeing. It says that children can tell the difference between a brand and a supermarket own version of the same product by the age of three. These children cannot read, so it is the images and logos that they recognize.

Mind maps are pictorial ways of organizing your thoughts. Some writing is used, but a mind map allows you to see clearly how one idea connects with another. Doodles are another visual way to unlock the thinking process. In this book, the 'Time for reflection' and 'Search and explore' action points are all illustrated by images which show you as the reader exactly what task you are being asked to do.

Reflection by doing

Sometimes, rather than talking it is better to 'do'. This is often true in group reflective sessions without a leader, where time can be lost talking and trying to define individual positions.

Most people have experienced a time in their lives when they have been able to have a difficult conversation with someone else precisely because they were doing something else. An example of this is driving, when people find it easier to talk intimately because they can't make eye contact with one another and are sitting beside each other rather than face-to-face.

Art therapy is a common practice in which clients are encouraged to draw, paint or mould a piece of work in response to what is troubling them. Usually in group reflective sessions there is no time to spend painting or drawing, and often people feel too embarrassed because 'I'm not a good enough artist' to work in such a way in a group.

One way of overcoming this problem is to use collage. A collage can consist of all sorts of things – you might want to use images, or words, or found objects. Any of these can be used to create a piece of work which gives you a picture of what you are reflecting on.

You might be trying to discover why something is making your group feel un-easy. At this stage, whatever is going on is one of those 'just a feeling' things for which you can't find words.

EXERCISE

Shared feelings collage
For this exercise, you will require some large sheets of paper, old magazines and colour supplements, scissors, marker pens, glue sticks.

Every participant takes a sheet of paper, on which they are invited to arrange images and words that apply to the way they are thinking about the problem the group is trying to solve. This doesn't have to be literal. If someone is feeling angry, they don't need to write 'ANGRY' in big red letters and find a face with a wide shouting mouth. Anger could be expressed by tearing things from magazines instead of cutting them or folding things tightly because they dare not let their feelings out.

Allocate ten minutes to this part of the session. When the time is up, ask the rest of the participants to look at all the pieces of paper and what is arranged on them. Do this in silence. When everyone has looked at everyone else's work, put another piece of paper somewhere where everyone taking part in the exercise can see it. Now, with discussion, try to identify whether there are common themes between the first set of collages. Perhaps two people have chosen similar images or arranged things on the first piece of paper in a similar way.

Now transfer anything that seems a common theme to a new piece of paper. Do not add anything or any words that have not already been chosen. The idea of this exercise is to focus down and explore people's first and immediate reaction.

When you have decided on what is shared, you can stick it down. Finally, ask the group whether they think anything has been missed from the shared collage. This could be from their own collage or from that of a colleague. If there is something a member of the group thinks must be part of the final collage, let them add it and decide where it should be placed.

Once the group has assembled the final collage, take five minutes to move away from it. Go and get coffee or walk outside for a breath of fresh air – anything which means you put a little bit of time between working on the collage and looking at it.

Now return as a group and have a look at what you have turned your feelings into. Feel free to discuss it with the other people who have created it. It might be useful to look at it from different angles. Do your feelings or those of others change as you look at the paper from the side or turn it upside down?

Many groups find it useful to photograph their collage as a way of recording it. You are now going to try and take one image from the collage as your final point of reflection. Often, through working together to this point, people find it easy to identify one shared image. When a group cannot agree, this usually points to an underlying dissension between members. This in itself can be an important discovery, so don't feel that your reflection has not worked just because, as a group, you cannot agree. Being able to disagree about things but still respect each other's point of view shows valuable maturity and professional understanding.

If the group you have worked with meets on a regular basis, you might want to make someone responsible for looking after the final piece you have created together so you can re-visit it, and also as it can feel uncomfortable throwing away a piece of work that you know contains colleagues' deepest feelings.

Walking for reflection

In the past, walking played a much greater part in people's lives than it does now. For many religions, the idea of going on a journey such as the Hajj or a pilgrimage was a way for a believer to discover more about themselves and their relationship with their god. In Europe, one of the most popular pilgrimage routes still walked, by believers and unbelievers alike, is that to Santiago de Compostela. People say the experience changes them because it gives them a chance to think and take things at a slower (walking) pace in a very busy world.

We are not going to ask you to walk the Camino but it is possible to walk for reflection in your own environment. Unless we consciously try to break it, most of us are creatures of habit.

 TIME FOR REFLECTION

Think of the order in which you get dressed in the morning. Was it the same this morning as yesterday morning? And the day before that?

Most of us take one direct and familiar route when we walk to places. Our aim is to get there as quickly as possible; we do not want to be distracted or held up on our journey. The idea of walking for reflection is to free your mind and enable things other than 'busyness' to enter.

The poet Wordsworth regularly walked for miles when he was trying to work out his poems and what he wanted them to express. His poem 'Daffodils' gives an idea of what walking for reflection can do for a person:

> I wandered lonely as a cloud
> That floats on high o'er vales and hills,

When all at once I saw a crowd,
A host, of golden daffodils;
Beside the lake, beneath the trees,

Fluttering and dancing in the breeze.
Continuous as the stars that shine
And twinkle on the milky way,
They stretched in never-ending line
Along the margin of a bay:
Ten thousand saw I at a glance,
Tossing their heads in sprightly dance.

The waves beside them danced, but they
Out-did the sparkling waves in glee;
A poet could not be but gay,
In such a jocund company!
I gazed – and gazed – but little thought
What wealth the show to me had brought:

For oft, when on my couch I lie
In vacant or in pensive mood,
They flash upon that inward eye
Which is the bliss of solitude;
And then my heart with pleasure fills,
And dances with the daffodils.

For Wordsworth, something he saw on his walk gave him pleasure to which he can return again and again. But his ability to do this was because he noticed the daffodils in the first place.

Before starting your walking reflection, you need to decide where you are going to go. If you have not done a walking reflection before, it is a good idea to choose to arrive at a place you know and which is not too far away. If you have limited mobility, your walk might involve the help of a friend, or a wheelchair. Having a destination in mind will help you to focus on your walk as you will not keep wondering where you are going.

Warm and comfortable – are you ready?

Take a few moments to think of your reasons for doing the walk. These might be:

- to solve a problem
- to have time to think
- to spend time with yourself

When you are ready, set off. Walk slowly but with purpose. Notice things as you go. Let yourself focus on the things you see. If you find yourself particularly attracted to something, ask yourself why. Does the over-flowing litter bin remind you of your over-crowded mind? Perhaps a bird flying makes you feel you would like to be free. As you walk, be prepared to change course. Take roads and paths you have not taken before. Look up as well as down. Be conscious of noticing things that you have missed before as you have rushed by. Is there a date carved over a doorway? How long ago was that? How has life changed since then?

Often, when you concentrate in this way, you will become aware of your spatial relationship to your environment. Enjoy this. Feel what it is like to walk across the middle of a bridge. If you can, jump the last two steps down. Perhaps you always walk close to the wall – is this because you feel protected and safe by it? Or are you one of those people who walks in the road because you feel frustrated at having to negotiate your way round other people on the footpath?

The Native American / First Nation peoples reminded themselves of their journeys and mapped them by using a memory stick. This is a stick to which they attached things that reminded them of the path they had taken. A feather might indicate where they saw a bird, or a leaf might indicate where they had had to turn by a tree. We are not asking you to make a memory stick, but you might find it helpful to pick up things that you find on your way as reminders of where you have been.

When you reach the point for which you set out, take time to pause and think back over your journey to get there. Enjoy the sense of having arrived. Pat the statue or feel the wall of the building. Ask yourself what are the new questions you want to explore as part of the journey. When you have done this, set off back to where you started.

You might want to take the same route home. If you do, notice how things change when you see them from a different direction. Walk back on the opposite side of the street and look in different windows. You may decide you want to take a differ-ent route back and explore different things. Feel free to do this.

When you arrive back, have one more quiet moment of reflection to think where you have been and what you have thought. If you have collected objects on your way, this is a good time to look at them and think about why you have chosen to pick them up.

This form of putting bits and pieces together to help reflec-tion is seen in 'memory quilts'. Don't worry, we aren't going to ask you to sew! Those of you who have seen a patchwork quilt will be aware that the composition and putting together of what could be random pieces creates something warm and comforting.

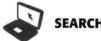 **SEARCH AND EXPLORE**

Try searching for The Names Project. This is a series of connected quilts that reflects on AIDS and those who have died of the disease. It is a piece of collaborative work by those who have shared experiences of a relentless illness.

Colours affect us

We all know that red is a sign of danger and that green means 'go'. Colour creeps into much of our language in the Western world: we are blue with cold and yellow-bellied with coward-ice. We are green with envy or pink with pleasure. Colour has a powerful impact on us and on our emotions (Craen, Roos, Vries & Kleijien, 1996). The authors show that patients taking placebos – these are tablets that look like the real thing but do not contain any of the drugs being tested – found the red, yellow and orange tablets were perceived as more stimulating than blue and green placebos which they found tranquillizing.

Colour is culturally defined; for example in Europe we associate black with mourning, whereas the colour of mourning in China is white. This means that reaction to colour is influenced by people's expectation rather than the colour itself.

If you buy clothes in big shops or over the internet, you are probably aware of the way a pair of shoes or a tee-shirt, though of exactly the same design, seem to be very different when seen in a different colour. Colour changes our perception of things and objects. In *The Mystery of Mercy Close* (Keyes, 2012) – a very funny, serious novel about depression – one of the ways the heroine's spiral into depression is depicted is through her admiration for paint colours with names like Gangrene, Poor Circulation and Frostbite.

 EXERCISE

With colours
Collect together seven pieces of paper in the colours of the rainbow, and a piece of white paper. Now, looking at the colours, reflect on an incident where you had a role that did not go as well as expected. Tearing or cutting the colours, arrange them so that they symbolize what you felt at the time. Now think back over the incident again and notice where you could have made changes which would have led to a more positive outcome. Space out the colours wherever you think you could have said or done something differently. These times when you could have made an intervention are represented where you see the white spaces between the colours.

Now look at the white spaces. What could you have done differently in the moment they represent? Perhaps you could have:

➤ altered your behaviour
➤ spoken to someone about the way their behaviour was affecting you
➤ taken a moment of calm by stepping out of a situation
➤ been more honest with yourself

Colour doesn't blame. But we can all beat ourselves up with words. Look at the white spaces and keep them as a reference for another difficult time.

EXERCISE

Using storytelling
This piece of reflection is designed to be done with a friend or colleague.

Sit down together somewhere quiet where you can listen to each other. Now tell the other person about a feeling you had as the result of something that has happened to you in practice: not the process, not the outcome, just the feeling and the events around it. Ask them just to listen and not interrupt until you have finished. This will probably take about two minutes.

Now let them share their feelings about an event with you. This time it is your turn to listen. You will probably find this difficult. Usually when we are with people we give them conversational prompts such as 'Then what happened?'

When you have both listened to each other, you are going to reflect back what the other person has told you. So if Malik told Sophie about his feelings of jealousy about someone getting a better mark, in the second part of the reflection Sophie is going to tell Malik how he felt. Again, it is important not to interrupt but to listen.

As you listen to your story back, you will want to interrupt and change what you are being told you said. Don't! Now tell the other person what they told you.

When you have done this, share what you feel about what you have heard both about yourself and about your colleague. Does hearing about your own experience from someone else help you to look at that experience differently? What has being in the role of a listener taught you? Did you share your feelings in an open and honest way?

Enjoying satisfaction

One of the ideas we have introduced you to in this book is the importance of reflection on things that have gone well. It is important to be able to recognize the sense of confidence and positivity that doing something well gives us. Identifying why something works and making it good practice leads to happier working environments than a culture which only reflects on things that have gone wrong. This final reflection without writing is designed to celebrate your reflective journey.

Enjoy it. Pleasure in doing things well is a valuable defence against the times when things go wrong.

EXERCISE

For pleasure
The ingredients you need for this reflection are:

➢ ice cream
➢ fruit
➢ nuts
➢ sprinkles
➢ chocolate

The equipment you need is spoons and tall glasses. You are now ready to make a Knickerbocker Glory based on the recipe of your reflection.

Method
Decide which of your ingredients represents the five components of reflective practice outlined in chapter 2. To remind you, here they are again:

➢ embed good practice
➢ record thinking process
➢ develop skills
➢ improve practice
➢ move difficult situations forward

Now make up your reflective treat by adding each of your ingredients in a quantity that seems proportional to your learning about *why reflect*. As with all

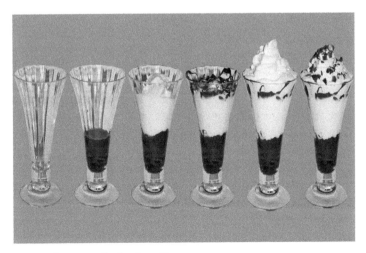

Figure 6.1 A Knickerbocker Glory

reflective practice, honesty and accuracy are important. If you have chosen chocolate to represent moving difficult situations forward but don't feel that you have understood this as well as you would like to, don't add more chocolate than you feel represents the situation.

Though everyone in the group will have had access to the same ingredients, everyone will have made a slightly different ice cream dessert. Celebrate what you have learned and eat your Knickerbocker Glory.

 EXERCISE

If you are interested in using non-verbal reflection in a care setting, we invite you to design and develop ways of reflecting that are appropriate for those you work with.

1. The Alzheimer's Society website has material on memory boxes for use with people in care homes. Using this research, can you develop your own memory box for those you work with?
2. The seminal work on how advertising works is *The Hidden Persuaders*, originally published in 1957 (Packard, 2007); this sits neatly with *Brandwashed* (Lindstrom, 2011). Reflect on how difficult it is to overcome the influence of commercial pressure, and the effect this pressure has on those with whom you work.

Summary

This chapter has made several suggestions for reflecting without writing, including the use of new media. We hope it has given you the confidence to try to invent different ways of doing this. For example, if you were celebrating the introduction of a healthy eating programme, making a Knickerbocker Glory would be completely inappropriate, but you could make a fruit salad and share that.

Perhaps because of the weather or your culture, going for a walk on your own is not appropriate – in that case, you could carry out a similar progress through your own home or even your own room.

Suggested reading for this chapter

We do not have any particular reading to suggest for this chapter. We hope that the sketch of digital developments has whetted your appetite for exploring these, and that we have given you sufficient pointers to explore a route that you are interested in.

Mostly, we hope that you will experiment with some of the ideas for non-written reflection we have given you here, and invent more of your own.

CHAPTER SEVEN

Reflective practice is ethical practice

Chapter Summary

This chapter explores in more depth the range of ethical issues related to reflection, and the ways in which practising reflectively can help in unravelling dilemmas. It will take the Neo-Aristotelian stance introduced in chapter 1 to look at issues of personal morality and will use reports of conduct hearings published by professional bodies and licensing authorities. These will be used to explore and critique situations in which practical wisdom is needed and to look at how reflection may help. Using the Reflective Timeline, it will 'unpick' the moment when the first bad decision was made and how that event was compounded by others. This chapter will develop your analysis beyond your own immediate practice. Through studying this chapter and engaging in the exercises, you will be able to:

- reflect on ethical dimensions of your own professional practice
- critically review your professional accountability
- develop your reflective practice to manage difficult situations

As you are reading this book, you are probably studying to join a health, medical or social care profession, or undertaking post-qualification study. In chapter 2, we said that reflective practice is useful for *improving practice*, and for *moving difficult situations forward.* We have then looked at the many ways in which you may reflect – alone and in groups, in writing and other media. We know that reflection is often hard; it may seem to be simply a chore that must be done, particularly when it's required to pass a course. We want to convince you that it is much more than that: a hard-wired way of thinking and behaving that sets you en route to being a successful professional.

We aim in this book to be positive and to encourage you to be courageous and confident in your skills. We want to show how, no matter what may go wrong – even if it makes you question your own abilities or threatens your career – reflective practice can be a helpful, essential life-line to ethical, professionally strong practice.

What does it mean to be a professional?

In chapter 2, we explored in detail different descriptions of professional behaviour (Litchfield et al., 2010; Pau & Croucher, 2003), but what does this mean to you? Being called a 'professional' may simply identify whether a person is paid or not – such as amateur and professional sportspersons. However, for health and social care professions, the distinction historically has usually been between 'profession' and 'vocation'. Many medical practitioners were not paid for their services and social or health care was provided by religious orders or by women who did so from religious conviction rather than to earn a living (Hallam, 2000; Hudson Jones, 1988). This left a cultural legacy that views engaging in caring work for money as less worthy than doing so because of a vocation. People reading this book will most likely share many of the ideals held to be vocational – for example, a belief that their work is worthwhile and that it is of value beyond the salary that can be earned. However, for the vast majority of you, your profession will be important to you not just as a worthwhile occupation, but as your source of financial stability.

Thus, to be a professional today usually indicates that

someone is at a particular level of skill, or capability. If you hire a professional to do work on your house, for example, you expect them to do a 'good job'. So a social care or health professional needs to be able to do well whatever aspect of care for people they are engaged in.

Professional status related to these behaviours brings with it privileges, but also duties. Privileges may include better salaries and conditions of work, as well as being held in higher regard than the average member of the population. Such status is also often associated with privileged rights to information, for example confidential facts about a person's life or their health status. Finally, it may permit you to undertake specific tasks. Examples might be prescribing and/or administering medicines; the completion of medical or other procedures; the implementation of legal acts that control behaviour related to mental or public health, and the safety of vulnerable children and adults (Purlito, 2011).

Duties clearly follow from this: if you know something confidential about someone, you need to keep that information to yourself, not to share it with others who do not have a right, or need, to know. If you have legal powers to restrict someone's freedom, or to prevent them from caring for their own children, your assessment of the situation must be absolutely clear and fair. If your professional status allows you to do anything to people's bodies, from requesting access to their homes or touching them to give care through to prescribing medications and carrying out invasive procedures, you have a duty to know what you are doing and the best, evidence-based way to proceed (Beauchamp & Childress, 2013; O'Hagan, 2007). These privileges and duties are more significant for professionals who have power and control over others: whilst you would expect the person who mends your roof or cooks a meal for you in a restaurant to be trustworthy in doing their job well, the level of their ethical integrity will probably be of less significance to you than for the person who is responsible for the wellbeing of your child or elderly relative.

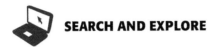 **SEARCH AND EXPLORE**

A search for 'professional rights and duties' will bring forward a wealth of material on this subject; you might want to narrow this down to look at aspects relevant to your country or profession, including human rights acts and other legislation.

Regulating the professions

Such freedom, power and responsibility means you are held ethically and legally accountable to a higher level than the average person. You are subject to additional laws, including the registration or licensing of your profession within your own country. The specific ways in which you are legally accountable will vary depending on your profession, your level of practice and the country you are working in. However, a useful overall guide to accountability is offered by Dimond (2008), who outlines the four arenas of accountability that apply to all (see figure 7.1). In this chapter, it is the fourth level – accountability to your profession – that will be the main focus for reflection.

Accountability

Accountability to criminal law includes serious crimes such as assault or murder.

Accountability to civil law includes, for example, disputes around negligence or breaches of privacy and confidentiality.

Accountability to your employer includes your contractual rights and obligations as an employee. This might, for example, include expected behaviour and confidentiality. It may include a 'gagging' clause related to whistle blowing.

Accountability to your profession for registered or licensed practitioners – this is an additional level of accountability that governs your behaviour. By accepting the privileged role of your profession, you also accept this set of added expectations.

Figure 7.1 The four arenas of accountability (Dimond, 2008)

Regardless of which profession you are studying to join, or already practise, the registering or licensing body in your home country, state or area will carry with it a code of practice.

 SEARCH AND EXPLORE

Do you know your Code of Practice? Find the site for the body that regulates and licenses your profession. Your Code will be published there. Bookmark this as you will need it regularly!

Have you found your Code? Whilst each profession may vary, there are three universal aspects.

(1) *To protect the public from harm*: for example, from physical danger, from breaches of confidentiality, from theft of their belongings or from poor practice.

(2) *To protect the good name of the profession*: each profession wishes to be held in high regard and to be respected by other professions and by the public. Someone who, for example, steals, cheats, or treats members of the public or other colleagues badly will cast doubt over the quality of the whole profession if this behaviour is not questioned.

(3) *To set standards for that profession*: Codes generally set out clearly what is expected of each professional. This Code then becomes the benchmark against which each person's behaviour and actions can be measured

The practical skills and knowledge expected will be different for each profession. The burden of responsibility for protecting and safeguarding children is present for all health and social care professions, but a higher level of knowledge, skills and responsibility may be expected for children's nurses, for midwives or in social work. A pharmacist or a doctor will have specific aspects of the management of medicines as part of their Code which would not be applicable to those working in social care. Despite these variations in detail, universal behaviours can be identified.

Research undertaken with medical doctors in Australia (Rogers & Ballantyne, 2010) looked at definitions used and, analysing them against decisions made in professional conduct inquiries, identified four features they claimed defined professional behaviour (p. 250):

- responsibility
- good relationships with and respect for patients
- probity and honesty
- self-awareness and capacity for reflection

These have a strong ethical bias and so seem to be a good summary of the universal nature of professional responsibility, harmonizing with the 'professional wisdom' of ethical practice (care, respectfulness, trustworthiness, justice, courage and integrity) introduced in chapter 1 (Banks & Gallagher, 2009).

What happens if you break your Code?

To illustrate the link between ethical professional practice and reflection, we will be using published cases, rather than the narrative stories we have constructed in other chapters. Our seven case studies are drawn from different regulators in Britain, Australia, New Zealand and Canada, and they concern people registered with seven different professions. (These countries were chosen because they publish more detailed accounts of cases, offering a more complete narrative. Other countries only publish the name of the professional, what they have done and the outcome – this means that it is not possible to have any insight into their feelings and motivations, or what might have influenced the decisions made regarding their right to continue practising their profession.) You will see that the mistakes they made, and the way their profession investigated and sanctioned their behaviour, are universal. In all seven cases, the allegations about them were upheld and their practice was limited or controlled as a result. As you will see if you search for cases from your profession, names are published, but we have chosen not to leave the actual names in the case studies we are using.

Anyone can contact your registration or licensing authority, reporting behaviour that they think falls below the standard for your profession. This can be anything from a formal police report when a major crime has been committed, through to an individual member of the public saying that you have treated them unfairly or dangerously. The allegation will always be investigated, and if your profession thinks that there is a case to answer they will hold a hearing. Unless the poor practice is related to a health problem, hearings are usually held in public and the outcome is reported openly on the internet.

The panel hearing your case will first decide whether the facts are likely to be true. If they are, then they will next make a judgement about whether your behaviour casts doubt on your worth as a professional. Finally, they will decide on what should happen next. Their job is not to punish, only to act in a way that will protect the public and maintain confidence in your profession, so they can choose to take no further action, caution you, impose conditions on your practice, suspend you from practice for a limited period of time, or remove your right to practise altogether.

Their decision will be made on the basis of the seriousness of the allegations, anything that you have done to show that you have improved your practice, and your insight into the issues raised by the allegation.

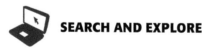 **SEARCH AND EXPLORE**

Did you bookmark your regulator's website? Go back to it now and find reports of completed hearings. The detail you are given varies from lengthy legal reports to brief summaries, but in each case the allegation, decision and outcome are given.

Through exploration of these cases and their outcomes, we hope that we can illustrate the ways in which reflective practice could, and in some cases did, help the practitioner concerned to understand and overcome their difficulties.

 EXERCISE

Before you read through the seven case studies, get your note book or sheet of paper, and create two columns like these:

What are the professional/legal issues?	What actions helped or hindered the practitioner's management of the situation?
•	•
•	•

Jot down the points that you think are significant as you read through them.

Case study A

A is a speech and language therapist working in the United Kingdom. He was investigated by the Health Care Professions Council, which regulates a large number of allied health professions and social work.

The allegation upheld against him included a range of issues:

That he was poor at managing his workload – for example time keeping, his waiting list and record keeping; the notes he did keep were just not good enough – they were incomplete and did not demonstrate that he knew what he was doing and was a safe practitioner;

that he did not respond to supervision and management by
following reasonable instructions or improving his practice; he
communicated poorly with colleagues and with the people he was
treating;
and that he demonstrated 'limited reflective ability' in that he did
not realize that his knowledge and abilities were below standard,
did not recognize that he needed help and did not improve his
practice.

The panel hearing this case was presented with no mitigation
by A, and with no evidence that he understood the issues being
raised or had done anything to improve his practice.

They made the decision to give a 'conditions of practice
order' – this meant that, in the present circumstances, he could
not practise, but, if he wished to return to his profession, he
could complete a remedial course and have his registration
reconsidered.

Case study B

B was a pharmacist working in Australia. All health professions have privileged access to restricted materials and
information, and in the case of pharmacy this includes drugs
that are only accessible on prescription.

One day B entered into an agreement to give some drugs to a
member of the public in exchange for money, without following
the legal procedure. This became a regular occurrence over several
years; B 'sold' increasing amounts of the drug to this person
without any regard for their health, or what they might be doing
with them. None of this was discovered until the person became ill
and was hospitalized.

Because B was accountable to Australian laws, as well as
to his profession, he was first tried and convicted in the local
courts. Following this, the Pharmacy Board of New South Wales
investigated his case. B did not come to the hearing or offer any
explanation of mitigation. Having been convicted, the allegation
against him was upheld.

*They made the decision to remove his registration so that he
could no longer practise as a pharmacist.*

Case study C

C is a physiotherapist working in Canada. The Canadian
health insurance system means that part of his practice is veri-
fying and signing for the treatment he has given or for special
aids made for the patients whose conditions he diagnoses and
treats.
*The allegations against C are that he has been filling in
documentation falsely, which has led to the insurance company
paying more than was needed. In addition, his record keeping
was poor.*
*It is unclear from the reports whether the lack of record
keeping was an indication of poor care given to his patients,
due to a lack of attention to detail or simply a way of disguising
the discrepancies between the care and treatment given and the
money claimed.*
*The disciplinary committee removed C's right to practise
for twelve months, but suspended this for six months during
which C had to submit to regular supervision of his practice,
unannounced inspection visits and detailed scrutiny of all his
records. He also had to install a computerized record keeping
system and pay hefty fines. Finally he was not permitted to act as
a supervisor of trainee practitioners.*

Case study D

D is a slightly different case of an English social worker, as
this was an incident that was nothing to do directly with her
practice.
*D drove her car having drunk considerably more alcohol than the
legal maximum. She was apprehended and convicted of a drink-
driving offence.*
Having been convicted, the case was referred to the Social

Work Regulator. Whilst no one was harmed, they concluded that it 'was behaviour that fell below the standards to be expected of social workers and had a tendency to bring the social work profession as a whole into disrepute. It calls into question her suitability to remain on the register.'

Because D admitted the offence immediately and had taken action to deal with her alcohol issues, the Council imposed an 'admonishment' (caution) to remain on her records for five years, but did not restrict her practice.

Case study E

E is a nurse who was taking a post-qualifying course that permitted him to be licensed to prescribe drugs. In the UK, this ability has now been extended to many health professionals but requires a post-graduate course and is strictly regulated.

Under pressure, due to problems outside work, E did not correctly complete all of the assignments needed to demonstrate he was safe to administer drugs, and falsified the evidence he had to submit to his university in order to qualify. He also handed in a portfolio containing plagiarized work.

E admitted that he knew at the time this was a dishonest and wrong thing to do.

The panel agreed that E's fitness to practise was impaired and suspended him from practice for four months.

Case study F

F is a doctor from New Zealand who failed to gain proper consent to do surgical procedures and then also failed to carry them out adequately and safely.

Although no fatal mistakes were made, these failings were serious, they did not occur just once and had affected patients and their families.

The panel reviewing his case noted that: 'He had been practising

*under supervision for a year at the time of the hearing and had
displayed an ability and genuine willingness to learn from his
mistakes and accept re-training.' They also noted that he had
suffered severe financial hardship (because he was not allowed to
work whilst awaiting the decision) and that he was insightful and
aware of his shortcomings.*

*They issued a formal 'reprimand', required him to continue to
work under supervision and imposed a fine.*

Case study G

G is a UK dentist who was investigated after being secretly
recorded in a television documentary in which she gave
misleading advice to a patient about treatment – in particular,
indicating that treatment provided by the National Health
Service (which is cheaper in the UK than private treatment)
would be inferior, when in fact the standard and materials
would have been the same.

*The dentist fully admitted the misconduct and was reflective
about the shame brought upon the profession and the
inappropriate discussion, which could have led the patient
to spend more money than was needed and to believe untrue
information about NHS care.*

*The misconduct was seen to be careless, rather than deliberate,
and the panel took into account insight and efforts made to
remediate. Thus a reprimand, rather than a more serious
penalty, was given.*

 TIME FOR REFLECTION

Think about your own practice for a minute. How close have you got to
situations that might have led to an investigation? What temptations or
difficulties in your own life might make you vulnerable?

Reflecting on the seven real cases, your table of issues and
actions may look like this:

Table 7.1 Case studies: issues and actions

What are the professional/legal issues?	What actions helped or hindered the practitioner's management of the situation?
• B, C, E and G were all dishonest	• A lacked realization/insight that there was a problem that urgently needed to be sorted out
• A's practice was poor and F's practice dangerous	
• B and C stole from others and G could have led someone to spend more money than they needed to	• A, B and C offer no explanation, and do nothing to try to make amends
• B, C and E forged documents	• D, E and G are honest about what they have done
• A, C and F were poor at record keeping	• D, F and G are insightful and take active steps to make amends
• B and D broke the law	
• All of them had poor judgement	
• All of them put other people at risk	
• All of them behaved in a way that questioned their fitness to practise	

In several cases, they have broken the law as well as their employment contract and professional Code – i.e. theft, fraud and driving under the influence of alcohol. You may have been surprised to see two cases where there was no direct link with professional care. Most professions take a poor view of behaviour that might reflect badly on them and will investigate any conviction, even if not related to actual practice. Investigations involving cheating in order to gain professional qualifications are a new trend, but case E is not unique. There is huge pressure on professionals to keep gaining more qualifications at higher academic levels. To protect the public and ensure professional standards are maintained, any attempt to acquire them through cheating and fraud is severely censured.

Reading through these cases you can see how easy it is, once something has started to go wrong, to end up in a really bad situation. None of these are evil people: they were not cruel or violent towards the people they cared for, but their standards were not good enough. All seven lack in some way the four behaviours identified in chapter 2 (Rogers & Ballantyne, 2010), and did not exercise practical wisdom (Banks & Gallagher, 2009).

You may particularly have noticed that lack of insight and reflection was noted as an additional issue in case A, and that D, F and G's prompt admission and actions to deal with their problems significantly raised the panel's opinion of their ability to continue to practise professionally. We want to suggest that learning to make some simple reflective behaviour an automatic part of your practice could avoid you getting into bad situations and help where you have a problem with your practice.

▶▶ *Stop before you start*
▶▶ *Know your weaknesses and limitations and get help*
▶▶ *Take action*

▶▶ Stop before you start

Imagine you can stop the pharmacist in case study B just at the point that the first prescription is illegally exchanged for money: a quick round of 'What? So what? Now what?' (Driscoll, 2000) (see chapter 2 for more detail on this model) zeroes in on the issues immediately.

> *What?* B has spent several years training to be a pharmacist and getting registration. He has the right to order, prescribe and handle drugs, under licence, that are not available to the general public. He knowingly gives restricted drugs to someone, not because of medical need, but because the person is paying him.
>
> *So what?* He is breaking the laws of the country he works in; he is taking no interest in, and showing no concern

for, the health of the person he is selling the drugs to, or the unknown other people to whom these drugs may be passed on; he is showing himself to be someone who is unprofessional.

Now what? Once the first transaction is made, he is in a difficult situation. With every prescription he illegally provides, he gets deeper and deeper in trouble.

The same is true for all of the other cases. Schön's 'reflection in action' (Schön, 1991) would have helped the physiotherapist in case study C and the nurse in case study E to think about the consequences of their actions. It seems clear that the doctor in case study G knew he was not gaining consent, and that the dentist in F was aware that her comments about poor standards of materials within the NHS would make her patient feel unsafe, for no good reason. An internal voice saying 'What are you doing?' could have stopped them. A moment's reflection, as illustrated by the Reflective Timeline, introduced in chapter 2, would have alerted them to the threat from their behaviour, to themselves and others. In all cases, this was not a heat-of-the-moment action; they all made a deliberate, conscious decision over a period of time to act in a particular way.

▶▶ Know your weaknesses and limitations and get help

No one is perfect; making a realistic honest self-assessment is a very useful skill for any professional, and reflective practice is a useful tool for developing this. The Reflective Timeline would call this 'Looking back' and 'Looking again'. In all seven case studies, there is a point where the person could have realized they had a problem and needed help. In each example, you can see a number of moments where their action negatively affected what happened next. Using Critical Incident Technique to deconstruct these moments is a way of understanding them better and seeing what might have helped to avoid a professional investigation.

Imagine the professionals in the case studies had used a Critical Incident Technique.

For example, in a supervision session, A is confronted with questions about his practice. The evidence is that record keeping and time keeping are poor.

What was critical? A's behaviour was having direct consequences for his patients – his waiting list was badly managed so people were not seen as they should be. His notes were poor so it was hard to tell whether the correct treatment had been given, and if anyone else had needed to take over they would not have known what he had done. A could have analysed the feedback. Why was this happening? Why now? There are so many explanations that we cannot know – he may have been ill, under huge personal pressure, feeling bullied and unsupported. Through being open to reflection, A could have identified the critical points, saving his career.

For D, being caught driving after drinking too much alcohol is her critical incident. Suddenly, a foolish act, caused by whatever distress was happening in her life at that time, is a potential threat to her career; she sees herself acting in a way that is not in harmony with the role and expectations of a professional person. Her response is to do things differently; the incident is a wake-up call that leads her to reflect on the problems she is having with alcohol and to do something about it. This case study also illustrated our third point: taking action.

▶▶ Take action

In all seven case studies, the way the person reacted to the investigation is very significant. We have deliberately not chosen the most sensational of cases reported, but even in a catastrophic situation where an error has led to death or injury, reflective practice can be a pathway out of trouble, a support through poor self-esteem, guilt and fear and into improved practice. Our suggestion in the Reflective Timeline is that 'moving on' is an important stage of reflection. This is when you take action and change your practice, but it is a frequently neglected aspect of reflection.

A had the opportunity to change through supervision, but did not – leading to the potential end of his career. B, C and E all took steps that led them deeper into trouble, thinking or hoping they would not be found out. The incidents relating to D, F and G shook the individuals concerned into taking action. This involved accepting responsibility for something that had gone wrong, identifying what could be done to make things better and acting upon this. Their actions made a significant difference to the professional investigation and its outcome. There are a number of key points that come from D, F and G's actions:

- making a mistake does not mean you are a bad person – you can have self-respect even if you know that you have done something wrong or foolish
- negative experiences are an opportunity to develop the practical wisdom necessary for the very best professional practice
- learning and moving on takes courage

Difficulties and limitations

 TIME FOR REFLECTION

All very well for you to say, you may be thinking: writing a book about reflection is a lot easier than being out there in the real, messy world. You may feel that you simply do not have the time to stop and think, that your circumstances are stressful, or your employment situation hostile and unhelpful. You may fear public exposure and may be hiding a lack of knowledge or ability. You may not feel very wise.

Reflection may cause you to challenge your own or somebody else's practice. Your reflection may show you that you have gaps in your knowledge and skills. Admitting this can be challenging but enables you to rectify the situation by asking for more training or reading up on the subject by yourself. What may be much harder is the realization you have identified poor practice in another professional; you have a responsibility to report this in an appropriate manner. Both these scenarios call for a degree of courage because they may threaten your relationships with others with whom you work, and your employment.

We are not saying that it's easy. These are all real barriers to reflection. In chapter 8, we look at circumstances in which you may have to face a challenging situation or report poor practice, and in chapter 9 we look at some of the difficulties with reflective practice.

The nature of reflective practice is that it is self-revelatory. It may cause you to reveal something about yourself and your past that you do not want to share. For example, you may find it difficult to behave professionally towards someone who arouses strong antipathy because of experiences from your past or because you have confidential knowledge about them that you cannot share with others.

Many writers struggle with these limitations – they want to portray reflection as a positive, life-affirming process – which it can be – but the reality for most people reading this book is that you will be being asked to use reflection as an integral part of your practice on the bad days as well as the good. At stages, before and after you are a qualified professional, you will need to use the medium of reflection and reflective practice to validate your professionalism and capability. Teasing out that which is yours – your own reflections and thoughts – from that which you share and exploring how they influence your practice and what you can do to overcome them is an important aim of this book. We all have certain prejudices but professionalism allows us to overcome these when working with clients.

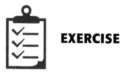

EXERCISE

You have already been through the process of thinking through an area of your own practice. Now try looking more critically at an aspect of your workplace, university or placement destination.

Find the policy for the area you are going to analyse that deals with disciplinary issues. Where are the opportunities for reflective practice to help you or others to navigate this policy? If you were asked to analyse it and offer improvement, what would you do to ensure that the organizational infrastructure enables and rewards reflection?

Summary

In this chapter, we have shown how reflective practice can be embedded into the way you think about and conduct your practice. Used in this way, it becomes much more than a tool for education, or for structuring an academic assignment. This is what it is really for and why it's worth making the effort to understand and practise the skills involved.

Suggested reading for this chapter

Beauchamp, T. L. & Childress, J. F. (2013). *Principles of Biomedical Ethics* (7th edn). Oxford: Oxford University Press.
Dimond, B. (2008). *Legal Aspects of Nursing.* Harlow: Longman.
O'Hagan, K. (2007). *Competence in Social Work Practice: A Practical Guide for Students and Professionals.* London: Jessica Kingsley Publishers.

Although written with different professions in mind, these three texts all explore professional behaviour and the boundaries of professional practice – for example, the explanation of accountability in Dimond has wide application, the cases in Beauchamp and Childress have resonance beyond medicine, and notions of competence that can be shared by all professionals working in this field.

Rogers, W. & Ballantyne, A. (2010). Towards a practical definition of professional behaviour. *Journal of Medical Ethics, 36,* 250–4.

An interesting and well-researched paper on professional behaviour. It is worth reflecting on the extent to which this can be applied to your own profession, and where your practice differs from that of others.

Other reading for this chapter is to seek out your Code of Practice, plus the regulations for practice and the legal requirements for your profession.

CHAPTER EIGHT

Asking difficult questions – exploring reflection in challenging situations

Chapter Summary

We all avoid asking difficult questions because we might not want to hear the answer. This could be because it is a threat to us or because we might have to confront ourselves or others about their behaviour. Reflection can lead you to difficult questions which are hard to avoid. In this chapter we will explore how reflection can help you to make sure you ask the right difficult question, using safeguarding adults or children and whistle blowing as examples. Through studying this chapter and engaging in the exercises, you will be able to:

- recognize areas of practice where challenging questions may need to be asked
- analyse factors for effective management of concerns at work
- apply reflective practice to the safe management of difficult situations

Moving difficult situations forward is one of the key reasons that we identify for engaging in reflection. In chapter 7, we explored the ways in which reflective practice can help when you are focusing on issues that arise in your own practice. Reflection can help you to challenge and improve your practice. Your reflection may show you that you have gaps in your professional knowledge and skills which can be easily rectified.

What may be much harder is the realization that you have identified poor practice or a problem in your workplace or with a colleague, or when you are confronting a particularly difficult problem in your own work. This may be obvious to you as soon as you start to think it through, or emerge as you look at the assumptions behind policy decisions through use of a critical reflection model (Fook & Gardner, 2007; Smith, 2011).

You may have a professional and possibly a legal responsibility to report something that is concerning you in an appropriate manner. These scenarios call for a degree of courage and the sort of professional attributes we introduced in chapter 1 (Banks & Gallagher, 2009). This may be because taking action threatens your relationships with people you are responsible for or people with whom you work, and may even threaten your employment.

There are times in your working life when nothing is obviously wrong, work is getting done, all of the things you can measure and record add up, but there's a feeling that something is not right. The niggle might not be there all the time but it keeps coming back. You can use reflective practice to play the detective. We are going to use two examples to explore an issue of safeguarding and whistle blowing, respectively.

Safeguarding

A concerned neighbour rings you to say that they are worried because Brian, a vulnerable adult, has been seen out without a winter coat on a very cold day. You call to see him. When you go to visit him, things are different from when you last met. He says there is no tea or coffee to offer you, his hair hasn't been cut and he hasn't done any Christmas shopping. Normally, Brian copes well with the help of a part-time carer. He loves offering visitors a drink and likes to be smart. Christmas is his favourite time of year.

You think back to a year ago. What's different? He seems not to have any money. You start to ask him questions. He really

*likes his new carer and tells you that his carer has started taking
money out of the bank for him and doing the shopping so he
doesn't have to go out in the cold. When you ask him about the
tea and coffee, he says that his carer has told him that everything
has gone up so much he couldn't afford them last week. Normally,
Brian has been able to manage his money and most of his day-to-
day living well.*

*The trigger for your reflection is a concerned neighbour
who has taken the trouble of contacting you as a professional
who is responsible for overseeing Brian's care package. Because
someone has alerted you, you now have a professional duty to
respond to the situation. In the past, the neighbour has done
things for Brian and they are friends; you judge that their
concern must be real if they have come to you in your professional
capacity.*

Put yourself in the shoes of the professional visiting Brian:
what are your immediate concerns when you see him? Using
the Reflective Timeline (see chapters 2 and 3), your initial
thoughts about what makes this moment critical might include:

- someone who prides themselves on their appearance has
  not had his hair cut
- a sociable person has not been able to offer you a hot drink
  on a cold day
- someone who loves giving presents has made no prepara-
  tions for Christmas

Looking back at what you have learnt, your first analysis is that money appears to be going missing. The thing
that seems to have changed most is the fact that there is
a new carer. This is a challenging situation because, even
though you may immediately suspect the carer, there
could be other explanations and you have no evidence.
Although Brian is a vulnerable adult, you do not have the
right to access his bank details and he seems to be happy
with the situation.

You ask Brian how the carer accesses the money for groceries. He says he has given her his pin number and card because she told him that he could be attacked and robbed when using the cashpoint. You decide that you should talk to the carer. But this is a delicate situation; you can't talk to the carer without Brian present, you may be accusing her of theft and you may jeopardize the good relationship between them.

You are faced with an ethical dilemma, where you must choose between actions, none of which is obviously the best.

 TIME FOR REFLECTION

What professional and emotional skills will you need to help you to get to the bottom of this situation?
Write down the questions you think you would ask.

This is where reflective practice can really help, using Schön's reflection in action (Schön, 1991) to think on your feet, or the 'in-the-moment' stage of the Reflective Timeline, where you capture immediate thoughts and feelings.

Safeguarding practice and professional responsibility vary between nations so knowing your own area and limitations will be important. Everyone has a role to play: social workers in the UK, for example, have specific responsibilities (Mantell & Scragg, 2011), but reporting concerns is everyone's business. You will need to be using all of your professional knowledge: skilled communication and detailed understanding about what, in your professional sphere, to look for.

 SEARCH AND EXPLORE

Safeguarding practice varies greatly across disciplines and is influenced by national laws. In the UK, searching for the Children Act may be a starting point, or look for the laws regarding vulnerable adults. Government reports on high-profile cases offer insights into best practice in this stressful and complex practice area.

The ethical skills and wisdom identified by Banks and Gallagher (2009) will guide appropriate behaviour. Looking again, you can see that you are *caring* and *respectful* towards Brian but also towards the carer. Rather than jumping to conclusions, you act in a *just* and thoughtful way, gathering information without assuming you know the truth. This takes some *courage*, and a lot of professional skill. It helps that Brian's previous involvement with you means he knows you to be *trustworthy*, so you may be able to ask the difficult questions that others could not.

Possible conclusions

Perhaps the carer avoids meeting you. She has Brian's pin number and his card. You may want Brian to ring the bank and the police, but he may be very upset about the idea and believe the best about his carer. If the carer has been stealing the money, she realizes that the game is up and disappears. The account number is changed and Brian realizes that he was too trusting.

However, there might be a more innocent explanation. When you finally get to speak to the carer, you discover that Brian has put down a deposit on a holiday and there has been a temporary cash-flow problem. He left his coat at the travel agent and he couldn't remember where it was. They will collect it when they go to town to do some Christmas shopping and get Brian's hair cut with this month's money.

Cases where you suspect someone who is vulnerable is in need of safeguarding are always difficult. You need to be very careful and well prepared with your challenge, which might lead to the investigation of another professional or a family member. Getting it wrong may lead to a victim being left in a bad situation, or to someone who should be investigated being left in a position of power. Getting it right might save a life.

Recognizing that you are in a critical situation, analysing

the issues and taking your learning forward will help you to move on and to become a confident reflective practitioner.

Whistle blowing

'Not again!' you think, as you walk towards Mary's hospital room. This is the third time that you have needed to come to see Mary and found the antibacterial handwash is missing. You work your way back through the department until you find a handwash that is not empty, clean your hands and return to her bedside, ten minutes wasted.

The previous week you attended the departmental meeting and heard of the changes that are being made to local budgets and to targets. You mentioned the handwash problem and several colleagues offered further stories about shortages of this and other products. Your concerns were noted by the manager.

As you leave, you begin to reflect on your day. You are conscious of feelings of frustration and not being able to understand why basic safety measures are missing.

 TIME FOR REFLECTION

Stop reading for a moment and reflect on this scenario. You might want to use the 'What? So what? Now what?' cues from chapter 2 (Driscoll, 2000).

Do you recognize a scenario like this? Is it familiar? Can you recount a similar story? We would be surprised if you have never been in a situation like this and cannot relate to the frustrations of working with limited resources, or of your concerns seeming not to be listened to or acted upon.

What? You felt frustrated and angry. You had to waste time that you could have spent more effectively. You happened to be conscientious, and would not have approached Mary without cleaning your hands, but would everyone bother?

So what? A basic, simple safety process has been breached. Your professional role could be anything from a verbal exchange to performing an invasive technique – either way, the lack of handwash means that infection and cross-infection become more likely.

What would have been the consequence of not washing your hands? How many other people might you have had contact with? How many opportunities would there have been to pass infection from one area of the building to another?

Now what? You did clean your hands. You also previously reported the problem at a meeting, and ensured that someone in authority was informed.

Is that it? Is that as far as your responsibility goes?

Key information: what counts as whistle blowing?

We often associate whistle blowing with high-profile cases in which huge sums of money are involved, the public are at grave risk or lives are lost that could be saved. However, the small things, such as a lack of day-to-day resources, like the handwash in our example, also fit this description.

 SEARCH AND EXPLORE

There are many high-profile cases of whistle blowing, in health care, environmental situations and the world of finance. You will find many general examples if you search for 'whistle blowing' and add your country's initials. And, for the UK, look up 'the Francis Report', which remains high-profile.

'Whistle blowing' has become an internationally recognized phrase that usually refers to situations in which someone who is employed in an organization discloses something that is wrong to a person who has the power within the organization to do something about it (Miceli & Near, 2002; Skivenes

& Trygstad, 2010). At the more routine end of this definition, it could include anything from day-to-day reporting of
shortages, to accidents or near-misses. For other authors, the
definition is narrower – for example, Lewis restricts it to just
where serious wrongdoing is reported publicly (Lewis, 2001).

Skivenes and Trygstad offer a useful breakdown of the
various stages of reporting issues, from routine through to
extraordinary:

> *Normal* activity is defined as everyday discussions about
> issues and perceived wrongdoing, where problems are
> discussed, and usually resolved at a local level. Day-to-day
> discussions and team meetings might be an example of
> this.
>
> *'Weak' whistle-blowing* activity is defined as the reporting
> of concerns directly to someone in the organization who
> has the power to do something about it. This might be
> through a formal meeting where concerns are recorded.
> Many organizations have 'reporting concerns' or 'escalat-
> ing concerns' policies to direct employees.
>
> *'Strong' whistle-blowing* activity is where the reporting of
> concerns is taken a step further. Perhaps the person
> reporting concerns can see that no action has been taken,
> or that the very people who are doing wrong are the people
> they should report to. Some whistle-blowing policies will
> direct employees to a more senior person they can con-
> tact; in other cases, the person reporting may decide to
> contact directly the most senior or powerful person that
> they can.
>
> *External whistle blowing* is where the person reporting
> decides to tell someone outside their organization. Again,
> this may be because they have tried all internal channels
> and do not believe the issue has been resolved, or because
> they believe the most senior management of the organi-
> zation is unable or unwilling to change the situation.
>
> (Adapted from Skivenes & Trygstad, 2010, p. 1078)

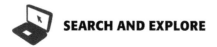

SEARCH AND EXPLORE

Your organization will have a whistle-blowing policy – it may be called 'raising and escalating concerns'. See if you can find it on your employer's systems, or your university intranet. Look too for advice from your professional regulator, union or an independent site offering support and legal guidance.

Why is it such a big deal?

This book is aimed at people from health and social care professions and we might think that all of the organizations we work for have the best interests of the public at heart, so whistle blowing should never be needed. A cursory look at newspaper headlines and recent history shows that this, strangely, is not the case. In the UK, high death rates for paediatric cardiac surgery continued for many years after an anaesthetist, Dr Stephen Bolsin, repeatedly called for reforms, and in the tragic case of 'Baby P' many opportunities to realize something was very wrong were missed, only to be exposed after the child died. The Francis Report (HMSO, 2013) has shown that, several years after both of the cases above were exposed, the same mistakes are happening. The prevalence of such cases, worldwide, shows that it is often ordinary professionals working in organizations who have to go to extraordinary lengths to get their voice heard to protect the people they care about.

Whistle blowing is a dilemma for professional people and a situation in which reflective practice can be crucial for several reasons:

- Your Code of Conduct will include a duty of confidentiality respecting the privacy of a person you are responsible for. How do you respect this when you report something that exposes their personal details?
- Your Code will include a duty of care: that you do everything in your power to ensure the safety and wellbeing of those you are responsible for. You will also be expected to work as

a team, and show loyalty and support for your colleagues. How can you do both if a colleague is responsible for the wrongdoing? Which do you choose?

- You are likely to have contractual duties; there may be a gagging clause on your contract that prevents you from talking to anyone outside the organization about its affairs. However, your professional Code will require you to report unsafe practice. How do you do the right thing and keep your job?

What factors affect whistle blowing?

Miceli and Near (2002) (see figure 8.1) suggest five factors are important in understanding whistle blowing.

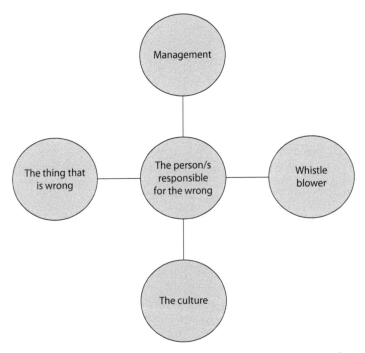

Figure 8.1 Factors affecting whistle blowing (adapted from Miceli & Near, 2002)

The thing that is wrong: how significant is this? It could be anything from a minor infringement of rules through to the embezzlement of huge sums of money or the endangering of lives.

The person/s responsible for the wrong: how powerful are they? Is it in their power to stop the wrongdoing? What do they stand to lose, or gain, if the wrongdoing continues?

The management: are policies in place that make everyone's responsibilities clear and encourage open behaviour? Are these policies mirrored in management behaviour?

The culture: what is the organization like? Do staff feel supported? Do they feel able to raise concerns?

The whistle blower: why whistle blow? And why now? Is the motivation personal responsibility, moral reasoning, malice, mischief? And do these motives matter?

Although Miceli and Near show the key factors involved, there is limited literature on what makes whistle blowing effective. Other research suggests that 'cost–benefit' analysis is something whistle blowers consider when deciding whether to report a wrongdoing (Somers & Casal, 2011). Others report that culture may also be important, as reported by Trongmateerut & Sweeney (2012), who explored differences between Thai and North American workers. These studies confirm that the interplay of the five factors in figure 8.1 seems to be important.

So, success is more likely where the solution is *easy to recognize*, staff that have the *power or authority to act* do so, and the *organization is open* to transparency and challenge.

Less success is evident where these factors are reversed, and/or where the wrongdoing is very serious. It may be that doing something about the wrongdoing will jeopardize the whole business, risking people's jobs. An example of this might be financial irregularities, or the recall of a faulty product. Another would be where the wrongdoers are very powerful people, who can threaten the whistle blower's job, or make their life miserable.

What happens to whistle blowers?

Sadly, the evidence is that whistle blowers are often treated very badly; your search of cases will have shown you this. Even where they are right, where there is legal protection and the issue is resolved, they may be bullied, and many leave their jobs. Worse still, many never see the wrongdoing corrected, or have to stand by seeing lives lost or endangered that could have been saved.

 TIME FOR REFLECTION

We offered a simple story of missing bacterial handwash to trigger your reflection earlier in the chapter. You may also have looked for some whistle-blowing cases on-line. If not, read the information box about Margaret Haywood (box 8.1). We are also sure that you will have a story from your own practice that illustrates the problems experienced by professionals when they are faced with shortages, poor practice or wrongdoing.

Using reflection to explore safely

We have seen that identifying safeguarding issues and whistle blowing both involve asking difficult questions and may involve making decisions with serious consequences; they can lead to personal worry, or the loss of one's job or one's livelihood. Despite legislation in various countries to protect whistle blowers, and legislation that requires professionals to report concerns, health and social care organizations have a very poor track record in supporting people who do so.

The Reflective Timeline (see chapter 3) can be used to establish the moments when a niggle or worry about something in your professional life will not go away, and to help you to manage these. By identifying critical incidence in your own practice and reflecting carefully and thoroughly, you can work out a course of action that has the most likelihood of success, at the least risk of damage to yourself or others.

EXERCISE

We will use the handwash example, and that of others such as Margaret Haywood, to illustrate this exercise, but you may well have an incident in your professional life that you are grappling with, or which has come back to you while reading this section.

In the moment: What exactly is niggling you? Be really honest with yourself! Write down the things that you think are wrong.

In the case of Mary's handwash, is it the risk to her safety and that of others that is uppermost in your mind, or is it that you are angry with management for making life difficult? You may have similar issues with the supply of basic safety equipment and feel angry and frustrated that such situations are allowed to happen.

Remember that the motivations of the whistle blower are often challenged. Indeed, some authors suggest that a person who reports wrongdoing out of malice or for their own personal gain may be dismissed as not a 'real' whistle blower (Miceli & Near, 2002).

Looking back: Why is this important? Try to think of all the reasons why it is important to reflect about this issue. You may want to think about it from the point of view of:

➤ The people who are users of the service: members of the public who may be reliant on help, or may be ill, frightened or disadvantaged.
➤ Yourself: how does this problem affect you, the work you do and your position in the organization?
➤ Your immediate colleagues: how do others feel about this? Do you talk about it? Have you tried collectively to find a solution, or do you feel that you cannot talk to anyone?
➤ The organization you work for: is it aware of the problem? How has it dealt with issues such as these in the past? What would be the consequences for the organization if the problem is not managed effectively?
➤ Your profession, the general public or other groups in society: perhaps there are also implications for them?

The lack of handwash for Mary is a serious issue. Hospital-acquired infection is a major source of morbidity, made more significant because it is usually preventable. Handwashing gel is one visible, simple way of reducing cross-infection, and increasing public confidence in safety.

All staff are put in a difficult situation when it is missing. You may be from one of a wide range of professions, either working within a hospital setting or responsible for visiting people when they are in-patients. You need to be able to get on with your job without delays, and to protect both the people you care for and yourself from infection.

The organization will be monitored: standards of hygiene and infection rates will be part of this. Outbreaks of hospital-acquired infections cause distress to the people involved, and also lead to financial losses.

Once you have analysed the situation from as many angles as possible, it's time to draw up an action plan.

Looking again: Bearing in mind the five factors in figure 8.1, can you draw up an action plan that is likely to be successful?

➤ Be very clear about what the problem is, and what needs to be done. Make sure that you know the facts and can verify them. Think about how and where you document this, referring back to the golden rules for reflective writing in chapter 4.
➤ Identify and follow the correct procedures in your organization for raising (and if necessary escalating) concerns.
➤ If your initial attempts to follow procedure and get something noticed or changed are unsuccessful, stop and think about why nothing is being done and what your next step is.

During your analysis, you will have reflected on the people involved and the sort of organization you work in. You may be raising an issue that could threaten the reputation of the organization, of your colleagues, or of someone senior and powerful; that could jeopardize people's jobs, including your own; and that challenges a particular deep-seated culture. This is where the dilemmas surrounding professional responsibility arise. You may want to talk to someone confidentially, using one of the websites you have found when searching for support. You may, like Margaret Haywood and others, feel that the injustice is so important that exposure to the public justifies the risk to yourself and the breach of the confidentiality of your organization.

Box 8.1 Margaret Haywood

Margaret Haywood is a British nurse who was so angry about the care of patients in a place she was working that she agreed to be an undercover reporter for the BBC and filmed poor care. Margaret was reported to the Nursing and Midwifery Council and struck off the professional register in 2009. This led to a public outcry and a systematic campaign for her reinstatement. Margaret appealed the striking-off order and was reinstated to the nursing register with a one-year caution.

Her case led to new policies and guidance across the sector, including professional regulators, unions and professional organizations and employers.

Whatever you choose to do, stop and reflect at each stage. The Reflective Timeline encourages you to 'look back' and 'look again', but then you need to 'move on' – making a decision and learning from your experience. You may come up with a clear strategy to whistle blow, but you can also decide that you can do nothing or seek a job in a different organization. This is your life and your career.

 EXERCISE

If you would like to explore this further, take the time to read Miceli and Near (2002) in detail. There is open access to the paper on the internet, so you should be able to find it through a simple search.

1. Thinking about the organization you work in (or another one that comes to mind that you are interested in exploring), and using the criteria Miceli and Near outline, identify the critical strengths and weaknesses that emerge.
2. If you felt the need to raise concerns, or to whistle blow formally, how easy would it be? What would be the barriers to your success and how would you try to overcome these?

Summary

In this chapter, we have illustrated two highly emotive areas of practice. Safeguarding vulnerable people and whistle blowing are issues that every professional will encounter at some time in their career. We hope we have convinced you that reflective practice is an essential element of your skill set when navigating this and other areas of concern in your practice.

Suggested reading for this chapter

Miceli, M. P. & Near, J. P. (2002). What makes whistle blowers effective? Three field studies. *Human Relations*, 55, 455–79.

Although this is now over ten years old, the model provided does not seem to have been bettered by later work, so is worth looking at.

Skivenes, M. & Trygstad, S. C. (2010). When whistle-blowing works: the Norwegian case. *Human Relations*, 63(7), 1071–97.

Much of the available research mentions cultural issues and this is the paper that makes them most clear. Worth reading and reflecting on, from your own cultural perspective.

We have not included any suggested reading for safeguarding, and legal issues and practice vary considerably between countries and professions. Your web search will have led you to legislation and practice that are relevant for you.

CHAPTER NINE

Is reflection always a good thing? Arguments and evidence

Chapter Summary

The title of this book is *Reflective Practice*, the length of it and the fact that it has been published implies that reflective practice is 'a good thing'. But we are sure that, on your journey through the book, you have had thoughts that reflective practice is not always the right practice at the right time. Your own experience may have shown you times when reflection did, or did not, help, or when you were frustrated by having to 'do' reflection that felt false or contrived. Our experience shows us that reflection can help individual professionals to develop, to manage crises and to improve the care that they give to others. However, reflection and reflective practice have little in the way of evidence of efficacy, or research-based validity, and, as we have discussed in chapter 8, there are times when it can lead to conflict and anxiety. Through studying this chapter and engaging in the exercises, you will be able to:

- critically review the case for, or against, reflection
- review some of the literature that explores the nature of reflective practice
- debate the issues raised when reflection is assessed

Are some people naturally more reflective than others? We have all said at some time: 'I wish I'd thought' or 'Why didn't you think?' These are expressions that we only use when something has gone wrong in some way. When some chance action has gone spectacularly well, we do not usually question it critically. Indeed, had the person stopped to think things through, the cat might not have been rescued or the football match won: too much reflection and thinking about things that could go wrong may stop us doing anything at all. We have all witnessed people who spend so long deciding what to do that in the end they do nothing.

Usually, when we do think before acting, we use our previous experience and our calculation of what could go well, or go wrong. How much we are willing to risk depends on how high the stakes are. A 20 per cent chance of winning a raffle may not seem good, but a 1 in 5 chance of an operation saving our lives may look like very good odds indeed.

In chapter 1, we introduced reflective practice as a technique that was developed as a counter to the 'technical rationality' of scientific methods of decision making, education and practice development in professions. However, its practical, 'messy' orientation makes it harder to research and less verifiable; the very reason for saying it's good makes it difficult to defend. Furthermore, embedding it into professional education has required assessment, usually through written accounts. How authentic are these? Do they truly 'test' how reflective the writer is or just how well they can 'play the game' and reproduce text in a reflective style? In this chapter, we want to focus down onto the three most difficult issues that we have come across in writing this book.

▶▶ Can reflection be taught, or is it simply more natural to some than others?

▶▶ Does reflective practice improve practice? Is there any evidence to support this?

▶▶ What are the issues with assessing reflective practice?

▶▶ Can reflection be taught?

We have spent a lot of time in this book trying to convince you that reflective practice is worth doing, that you should learn to do it, and strive to do it better. Is it something you can be taught – that through instruction, knowledge and skill acquisition can be improved and mastered?

Schön's argument, introduced in chapter 1, is that professional learning has come to rely upon 'technical rationality'. The educational process he challenges – of starting with rules and theory and moving on to practice later (Schön, 1991) – suggests that the basic rules of a task need to be taught and learnt prior to mastery and intuitive working. The reversal of this process in reflective practice – stating that the *practice* of a profession is where learning should start, with application and theory following from this – locates reflection in doing and being a professional, rather than thinking and reading. Edwards and Thomas strongly argue against reflection being taught: 'reflective practice cannot be a rubric of prescriptive skills to be taught. In fact, to view it in this way reverts to the very technisist assumptions reflective practice was meant to exile' (Edwards & Thomas, 2010, p. 404).

However, if reflective practice is something that we desire, and even require, from professionals, can we assume that they will automatically understand and be able to do it? Other authors (such as Russell, 2005) disagree, stating that it should and ought to be taught: how can we ask students to be reflective, tell them it is important and ask them to get better at it, if we cannot teach it? Some of his concern comes from reports he has heard from students that they make up stories for assessment, which suggests that teaching reflection needs to be seen in connection to assessing it, an area we discuss later in this chapter. He argues that students need to be given clear structure, and to be assessed, in order to frame and develop written reflection. Whilst he refers to teaching, what he describes may be closer to 'facilitated learning' (Bolton, 2012). This issue may be one of semantics, or the philosophical matter of the role of 'teacher' and 'learner' in an educational setting.

Although research evidence is limited, a literature review (Mann et al., 2009) sifted through hundreds of published papers to identify twenty-nine empirical studies exploring reflection in medical and nursing education. They judged these to be well designed and thorough, but mainly exploratory and qualitative in nature. Just four of the studies aimed to test whether reflection had been taught – these conclude that the studies did show a difference in students' reflective ability over time. However, the designs tended to rely on the assumption that the assessment of student learning is a measure of their increased reflective ability.

This assumption is supported in other studies, for example an experimental design with three groups attempting a written reflective assignment: a control group with no additional support, a group with 'critical incident prompts', and a final group with an additional flow diagram to aid structure (Lai & Calandra, 2010). They found that the two structured groups wrote better assignments, with more evidence of 'higher level' reflection. We would like to argue that studies claiming to show that reflection has been taught by measuring reflective writing may be oversimplifications. An alternative explanation for the assessment results is that students learn to demonstrate what is valued by the person doing the marking, rather than becoming more reflective.

A further study with medical and dental students (Brett-MacLean et al., 2010) claims that developing narrative reflective practice did help students to 'story' their own development and empathetic understanding of the people they were caring for, but, as with other studies, they fall short of suggesting that this, of itself, shows that reflective practice can be taught.

So can it? We recognize reflection and reflective practice in ourselves and others and often note an absence of reflection, which suggests that it has been learnt, but how and when that learning takes place, and the role of formal teaching and learning, are much less clear. What seems obvious to us is that it is not learned in a classroom, and is not learned just from reading about it. Things that seem to be important are:

- spending time thinking, returning to events and actions in order to appraise their meaning
- engaging in group or one-to-one dialogue
- recording reflections in some way – written or otherwise
- feeling safe to explore without being judged

Perhaps most importantly, these acts are undertaken in parallel with being a particular person, a combination of professional and personal identities. These are framed, or motivated, by a moral agency akin to professional wisdom (Banks & Gallagher, 2009) and values-based practice (Thornton, 2008).

▶▶ Does reflective practice improve practice?

It is clear from the research undertaken to identify how reflection is taught, and the experiences of trying to assess its existence and quality, that not everyone finds reflective practice easy, and many respondents in research and opinions in published papers challenge its worth. So why do it? Is there any evidence to support the role of reflection in improving practice? And if there is not, what is its purpose?

A number of papers report findings that claim a link between reflection and practice improvement. Mamede and colleagues argue for a relationship between being able to reflect critically on practice and the reduction in diagnostic errors (Mamede, Schmidt & Rikers, 2007). They identify that, whilst some errors may be unavoidable – for example, unpredictable factors or systems failures – many errors are cognitive. Their work is supported by later authors: firstly, Barley (2012), who accepts the theoretical position that managing complex cases is aided by reflection, but acknowledges there is yet to be robust research evidence to confirm this; secondly, Wald and Reis (2010), who reprise some of the arguments about how to assess through focusing on how to measure reflection from reflective writing. Both papers acknowledge that possible links between reflection and diagnostic reasoning cannot be assumed to be measured through reflective writing, and that formal assessment can lead to formulaic answers.

Similarly to Benner's 'expert' nurse (Benner, 1984), experienced doctors in Mamede's later work use pattern recognition and heuristics to fast-track decision making, thus creating bias that may miss important signposts to alternative decisions (Mamede, Schmidt & Penaforte, 2008). They identify a number of elements that are involved in reflection, concerning questioning, testing, exploring and being open to criticality and learning. Although empirical testing showed no statistically significant improvement in decision making, they did note that reflective skills were significant when dealing with more complex situations, echoing Schön's theoretical position on the 'messy swampland' of professional practice, introduced in chapter 1 (Schön, 1991).

Other authors note positive connections between reflection and practice improvement: Balla et al. (2009) and Graber (2009), looking at decision making for family doctors and clinicians; McCracken and Marsh (2008), focusing on evidence-based practice related to social work; and, looking at expertise in nursing, MacLeod (1996), who identifies that defining features of the experienced ward sisters in her research were *reflection* and *openness to learning*. By contrast, practitioners who were not judged to be experts by their peers lacked the critical awareness associated with reflective practice (Benner et al., 2009).

Research with students, using digital equipment to log encounters that included cues to record related learning points, found a correlation between the logging of encounters and therapeutic relationships, and also between logging and interpretation skills, but not increasing factual knowledge

(Thomas & Goldberg, 2007). Further evidence is offered by Glina and colleagues, who record the positive effect of group reflection on performance for a group providing hospital food services (Glina et al., 2011), and in research undertaken with nurse practitioners (Glaze, 2001, 2002), who identified (self-reported) positive responses to the effect of reflective practice.

So where does this leave us? Whilst much that is written about reflective practice is uncritically positive, there does seem to be a growing evidence base that supports the efficacy of such practice in:

- linking reflection with critical thinking skills and complex decision making
- supporting new people to learn and grow into their professional role, and experienced people to continue to learn and survive in complex and often stressful environments.

Many questions remain, not least of which are the relationships between personality and the tendency to be reflective, the role of culture and upbringing, and the extent to which innate learned behaviour and thinking can be directed, changed or improved through teaching or facilitated learning.

Finally, the results of empirical research are based on an assumption that we are able to identify what reflective practice is with sufficient clarity to measure it. This challenge is often mirrored by equally compelling issues regarding the assessment of reflection.

▶▶ What are the issues with assessing reflective practice?

Since the turn of the century, a growing number of papers have appeared challenging the validity of assessing reflection and reflective practice. They suggest that we are not confident we know what we are trying to assess or why, or whether the assessment tasks set measure or test the things that are being looked for.

A talk by 'looked-after' children (children who are brought up by someone who is not a member of their birth family) left two students with very different responses.

One student was horrified and angry that there was such a category as 'looked-after' children. In the culture from which she came, children who had lost their parents would have been taken in by a relation, however distant, and the concept of looked-after children simply did not exist. Asked to reflect on her feelings after the talk, the student could only write about the shock of discovering that the society in which she was studying could think it appropriate to treat children in this way.

Another student who had been present at the same talk was deeply surprised that the children had said one of the things they disliked was being taken by social workers to discuss their cases at a local fast-food restaurant. This student thought that the children were being ungrateful and that they should see being taken to the restaurant as a treat. The student was unable, as a single parent, to afford family outings to the same restaurant and so thought the looked-after children 'lucky' to be given treats.

After reflection, the second student could recognize that the looked-after children did not like to be seen by their friends with their social workers. It was not the restaurant they were objecting to but the fact that others at their school might discover the truth about their family background. The student's reflective journal was marked and passed.

The first student found it impossible to accept a culture that did not have strong kinship ties. The points she was making in her reflective journal were extremely valid but she was not able to debate her points within the structure required by the journal. Instead of an honest piece of reflection on herself and her response to the talk, she felt compelled to hand in a piece of work that was not honest to get the mark she required for the module.

TIME FOR REFLECTION

Stop for a moment to reflect on this story – a fictionalization of a real event. How do you view the two students? Is one 'better' or 'worse' at reflection than the other? If both views are valid, how would you 'grade' their reflections? What advice would you give the student who feels that she could not be honest in the assessment?

This story will be familiar to anyone reading this book who has been involved with being assessed, or with assessing reflection. Both students' reflections are valid and insightful. The facilitated learning has been effective as a trigger for greater understanding of the society in which they were learning to be professionals. Both have strong feelings that have led to reflection and learning. Should you judge them, and if so how? Is one 'more' reflective because they can articulate the process of learning to view the situation through the child's eyes? Is the student whose cultural values are offended 'less' reflective because she struggles to contextualize this?

Educational models such as 'constructive alignment' (Biggs, 2006) view assessment as an important, integral part of learning as well as a measure of attainment. First, 'learning outcomes' articulate the lecturer's aspirations for the changes in student knowledge, skills and attributes brought about by a particular course of study. This is then supported by a learning and teaching strategy that facilitates achievement of the outcomes. Assessment aligns with these processes to scaffold, measure and reward learning. Finally, feedback on student achievement and evaluation of the experience 'feeds forward' into ongoing student learning and curriculum development. The assertion that assessment is one equal component of this learning process is well established and accepted.

However, for all our belief that reflection is important to professional practice – that it can help to embed good practice, facilitate the recording of thinking processes, develop skills and improve practice and may help to move difficult situations

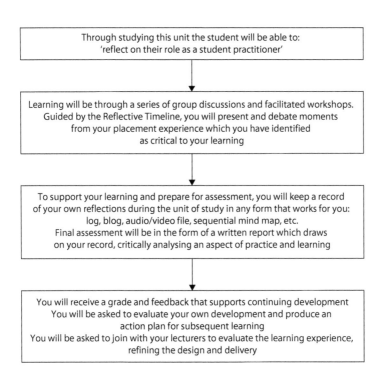

Figure 9.1 Flow diagram of a learning experience using constructive alignment (after Biggs 2006)

forward – we acknowledge that the role of assessment in this may be flawed.

A student following a course of study using constructive alignment (see figure 9.1) may be a wonderfully reflective practitioner, but we are not convinced that the assessment is a faithful and reliable measure of this. Students who have mastery of the written discourse of reflection may be able to write eloquent prose but this does not 'prove' their reflective ability (see chapter 4, where we demonstrate how to produce a reflective essay). The measurement of reflection through written artefacts is about demonstrating to a third party (the person doing the marking) that you (the student) understand the rules of your profession, which typically include recognition of the boundaries of acceptable and unacceptable practice and discourses about care, compassion and avoiding discrimination.

A growing literature explores the difficulties with assessment: that the narratives that may be perceived to be acceptable, and thus to get the best marks, are limited to those which tell stories of acceptable professional behaviour (Hargreaves, 2004). 'Eating humble pie' and 'toeing the line' (Macfarlane & Gourlay, 2009) may lead to conformist rather than thoughtful and critical enquiry, and 'strategic reflection' (Hobbs, 2007) may involve faking reflection. Barley refers to assessment as potentially 'a process of atonement rather than learning' (Barley, 2012, p. 277) and Ross alerts us to the additional challenges faced when reflecting in digital forms which add a new dimension of surveillance and control (Ross, 2011). Perhaps what all have in common is that students will inevitably learn to present and express their reflections in the way most valued by their lecturers, rather than in a way that is most helpful to their practice.

Other authors suggest that reflection for professionals needs to go further than personal introspection, looking critically at assumptions behind thoughts and feelings and the socio-political context in which the reflection takes place (Brookfield, 2009; Fook & Gardner, 2007; Smith, 2011; Thompson & Pascal, 2012). Doing this encourages students to look beyond their own experience.

 TIME FOR REFLECTION

Look back to our story of the two students and the looked-after children – how might a critical approach to reflection have helped them to explore the links between their own experience and that of the looked-after children talking to them?

In their review of the literature, Mann et al. (2009) ask whether reflective thinking can be assessed, a question addressed by nine of the twenty-nine empirical studies they identified. These studies support the idea that it can; however, they acknowledge that this assumes writing can be taken as proxy for reflection and that assessing 'writing' does not necessarily test or assess reflective practice. Although this review supports other literature, the authors highlight one particular dilemma by suggesting that, although there are limitations to assessment, *not* assessing may be interpreted by students as a lack of value being given to the reflective activity.

Research undertaking detailed discourse analysis of written reflection for assessment (Bos, van Opijnen & Zomer, 2012) concludes that, through textual analysis, 'reflection can be measured with elements that actually do predict "good" reflection' (p. 633). These authors are clear that aspects of the text do correlate with elements and stages of reflection. Similar methodology is used to deconstruct students' text in Wharton (2012) – this time involving individual reflection following group activity. Wharton's findings raise issues about truthfulness, how to present 'self' and strategic decision making about what to write. Both papers may reinforce the challenges to assessment presented above (Hargreaves, 2004; Hobbs, 2007; Macfarlane & Gourlay, 2009; Ross, 2011), as they indicate that learning to produce text that correlates with assessors' beliefs about what 'good' written reflection looks like may become the primary goal for students who wish to do well, rather than actual engagement in the reflective process.

These challenges give written reflection a bad name. Bolton (2012) argues that assessing students' reflective writing is not so much an act of testing their learning – it is more a matter of facilitating people being better at reflection *through* writing, which enables learning and change. Others suggest structures to aid assessment (Bourner, 2003) and various techniques such as learning journals and portfolios (Bulman & Schutz, 2008; Moon, 2006). It is clear from their extensive knowledge, and from our own experience, that writing reflection can be a very powerful medium for development and change, but from numerous papers there is compelling evidence that assessment and grading, particularly where these are directly linked to success and failure on a professional course, inevitably change the nature of what is written.

Learning and teaching activities that enable self-assessment are identified by Mann et al. (2009) as a possible solution. Carefully constructed and long-term research in collaboration with students may also be a way to identify successful strategies (Stewart, 2012), but even when we think we have got it right, the reflection may not be authentic from the student's perspective.

A number of key points emerge from this literature:

- Tasks with clear assessment criteria will guide students to follow them – so the quality of the 'reflection' will be determined in part by the quality of the learning outcomes and assessment criteria
- Reflective writing is a technique just like writing a report, essay or dissertation. We should not mix up good writing technique with good reflection
- But: helping students to communicate their reflection skilfully to others is worth doing
- And: nurturing reflective practice that is perceived as important and valued by students without formal assessment is difficult but essential.

So has this review helped? We remain convinced that reflection is important, that we have seen it, recognize its power and want to help health and social care professionals to achieve it. We hope that, by offering this critique of the pitfalls of assessing reflection, students and teachers can have a more honest and open debate about how and what to assess.

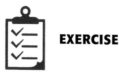 **EXERCISE**

In this chapter, we have offered a more theoretical view of reflection. If you are interested in pursuing this further, the literature here represents a fraction of the published materials available. Depending on which of our three issues you are most interested in:

1. Using one of the models offered in this book, make your own learning of reflection the focus of your thoughts. Can you identify the ways in which you have learnt to be reflective? Has 'teaching' helped, and if so how? Do you recognize your own experience in the academic papers discussed?
2. Identify the papers referred to here that claim a link between reflection and improved practice. Critically review the research design and methodology. Are they compelling? Do you trust the conclusions they reach?
3. Take a piece of your own reflective writing and two highlighter pens. Highlight the sections that accurately demonstrate your reflection (be honest! – no one is watching), and the sections that apply theory, analyse or critically analyse practice. How did you do? What was left after your highlighting and what was its purpose? Now think of a situation in which you feel that you were truly reflective: could you capture this in writing, or would another medium be better?

Summary

In this chapter, we have tried to address three of the issues that we have returned to regularly during the writing of this book. A common theme in all three questions – whether reflection can be taught, whether it makes a difference to practice, and whether we can honestly and accurately assess it – is the difficulty in defining and recognizing reflection and reflective practice. Understanding that reflection, like compassion and wisdom, is demonstrated through doing may be helpful in unravelling this problem.

Suggested reading for this chapter

Edwards, G. & Thomas, G. (2010). Can reflective practice be taught? *Educational Studies, 36*(4), 403–14.

One of the texts that critiques the 'teaching' of reflection. This sets out the arguments well.

Glina, D. M. R., Cardoso, A. S., Isosaki, M. & Rocha, L. E. (2011). Participatory ergonomics: understanding the contributions of reflection groups in a hospital food service. *International Journal of Industrial Ergonomics, 41*, 96–105.

This one is useful because it's a piece of real, empirical research that does seem to make links between reflection and performance in practice. Interesting, too, as this was a group reflection situation.

Biggs, J. (2006). *Teaching for Quality Learning at University* (2nd edn). Maidenhead: Open University Press.

A useful all-round text for curriculum design and development, and a good read if your role is in education.

Bos, J., van Opijnen, J. & Zomer, P. (2012). Are you talking to me? Assessing discourses on reflection. *Reflective Practice: International and Multidisciplinary Perspectives*, 13(5), 621–35.

This is one of the texts from educational research that deconstructs reflective writing. A useful read for critical analysis of assessing reflection.

CHAPTER TEN

Conclusion: embedding reflection – looking forward

Finding the honest route

This book has been written by authors from two very different backgrounds. Janet is an academic working in a university but her roots are in nursing. She has changed dressings and emptied bedpans. Louise is a playwright with an interest in science and medicine. We have both worked with students to help them to understand and improve their academic achievement and their practice. We both have experience of health and care services.

Janet's reflections on working on this book: This has been a roller-coaster ride for me. I trained as a nurse and had no idea I would ever be an academic in a university. Even though I have a doctoral qualification and I have published, I have never written a book before. I have taught and written about reflective practice for many years and have always been very sceptical about the way we teach and assess it. Writing this book has given me the chance to set out what I believe is a useful, achievable and ethically sound way for professionals to engage in reflection. Writing it with Louise has added dimensions that I would never have thought of on my own.

Louise's reflections on working on this book: Though I feel confident when working in the theatre or television, academic writing is very different. It requires a discipline and truth that I can't invent or 'improve' in the same way I can in fiction. Working with students I was shocked by how difficult they found reflective writing and how worried they were about being honest about their feelings when they knew their work was going to be seen by their tutors. One of the reasons for writing this book was to address this problem. I do a lot of my thinking while doing other things, which led to chapter 6, 'Expressing reflection in other ways'. My husband is disabled and I have been surprised by the lack of co-ordination and shared language between social and medical services. I'm used to writing on my own, and working with Janet has taught me a lot about collaboration and joint responsibility.

Our emphasis while writing this book has been on helping you find an honest way:

- to record your reflection truthfully
- to confront painful and difficult things
- to celebrate your success
- to work openly with other people

We hope we have succeeded.

Why reflect?

In chapter 2, we asked you: Why reflect? You will now have used the Reflective Timeline in a variety of situations. You have done individual and group reflection. We have encouraged you to consider inter-professional working relationships. You have written, thought, walked, talked and created in a reflective manner. The confidence and competence that can be gained from reflection will help your practice to be grounded and valuable for yourself, your colleagues and most of all, the people for whom you are responsible. So, looking forward, how can the five reasons we offer for engaging in reflective practice help you to become a trusted and focused professional?

Embed good practice

This allows you to trust your own judgement and make decisions based on experience as well as evidence-based knowledge. Because you have a body of knowledge and a method of thinking, you will also be able to respond to more unexpected situations by building on what you know.

Being a reflective practitioner (Schön, 1991) can be the key to your success. Through using the knowledge and theory embedded in your actions when you reflect in and on action, plus the personal attributes of care, respectfulness, trustworthiness, justice, courage and integrity (Banks & Gallagher, 2009), embedding good practice can become a reality.

Record thinking processes

You have learned the importance – personal, professional, ethical and legal – of recording your thinking as part of reflection. We have shown you that it is not always about writing – as long as you can return to what you have recorded and it has meaning for you, any process is valid.

There will be times, such as assessment and formal reporting, when written evidence of what you have done will be important beyond your own interest and achievement. But you now have a range of techniques which will help you to record in the professionally appropriate way. You no longer have to fear a blank screen or empty sheet of paper because you don't know how to start.

Believe us, we know how scary a blank screen can be, but while writing this book, once we had put down the chapter number and a line about content, we were able to move on fairly fast and fluently.

Develop skills

If you were completely new to reflective practice, you now have an understanding of the process and range of strategies. You know what a valuable tool it can be and may be using it outside your professional life to make decisions and clarify things.

If you were already a reflective practitioner, we hope that we have introduced you to new and different ways of reflection. Reflection is a means to an end and will have helped you to develop other skills. We have talked about inter-professional working relationships and demonstrated how reflection can cross professional barriers. This grounding will give you more flexibility within your career, enabling you to make informed choices about your working life and future.

Improve practice

We believe the confidence you have gained through your reflective practice will improve the lives of those you work with and are responsible for. We have experienced this for ourselves, and observed and worked with many people who report that their practice has been improved and enriched by reflection.

In chapter 9, we identified that many of the papers published about reflection are just examples and people's opinion. However, there is also a growing amount of recent research that shows reflective practice making a real difference when done well.

Move difficult situations forward

Your professional world won't always be full of success stories. When things go well, celebrate them! This will help you to be more resilient in difficult and stressful situations.

When your practice is challenged or you see something that disturbs and troubles you, we have demonstrated that reflective practice can be a vital key to unlocking the situation. It helps you to identify reality and find the courage to deal with problems. It could save your career or someone's life.

Summary

As we come to the end of the book, we want to remind you that reflection is a sensory, emotional process. Capturing the moment, but then spending time using your senses and intellect to learn, develop and move on, will mean you complete the Reflective Timeline, and use it to support your practice and your life.

References

Arber, A. (2006). Reflexivity: a challenge for the researcher as practitioner? *Journal of Research in Nursing*, 11(2), 147–57.

Balla, J. I., Heneghan, C., Glasziou, P., Thompson, M. & Balla, M. E. (2009). A model for reflection for good clinical practice. *Journal of Evaluation in Clinical Practice*, 15(6), 964–9.

Banks, S. & Gallagher, A. (2009). *Ethics in Professional Life: Virtues for Health and Social Care*. Basingstoke: Palgrave Macmillan.

Barley, M. (2012). Learning from reflective practice and metacognition – an anaesthetist's perspective. *Reflective Practice: International and Multidisciplinary Perspectives*, 13(2), 271–80.

Beauchamp, T. L. & Childress, J. F. (2013). *Principles of Biomedical Ethics* (7th edn). Oxford: Oxford University Press.

Benner, P. (1984). *From Novice to Expert: Excellence and Power in Clinical Nursing Practice*. Menlo Park: Addison-Wesley.

Benner, P., Chesla, C. A. & Tanner, C. A. (2009). *Expertise in Nursing Practice: Caring, Clinical Judgement and Ethics* (2nd edn). New York: Springer Publishing Company.

Biggs, J. (2006). *Teaching for Quality Learning at University* (2nd edn). Maidenhead: Open University Press.

Bolton, G. (2012). *Reflective Practice: Writing and Professional Development* (3rd edn). London: Sage Publications.

Borton, T. (1970). *Reach, Touch and Teach*. London: McGraw-Hill.

Bos, J., van Opijnen, J. & Zomer, P. (2012). Are you talking to me? Assessing discourses on reflection. *Reflective Practice: International and Multidisciplinary Perspectives*, 13(5), 621–35.

Bostridge, M. (2008). *Florence Nightingale: The Woman and Her Legend*. London: Penguin Books.

Bourner, T. (2003). Assessing reflective learning. *Education and Training*, 45(5), 267–72.

Brett-MacLean, P. J., Cave, M. T., Yiu, V., Kelner, D. & Ross, D. J. (2010). Film as a means to introduce narrative reflective practice in medicine and dentistry: a beginning story presented in three parts. *Reflective Practice*, 11(4), 499–516.

Brookfield, S. (2009). The concept of critical reflection: promises and contradictions. *European Journal of Social Work, 12*(3), 293–304.

Brown, A. D. (2010). Social media: a new frontier in reflective practice: commentaries. *Medical Education, 44.*(8), 744–5.

Bulman, C. & Schutz, S. (2008). *Reflective Practice in Nursing.* Oxford: Blackwell.

Butterfield, L. D., Amundson, N. E., Maglio, A.-S. T. & Borgen, W. A. (2005). Fifty years of the critical incident technique: 1954–2004 and beyond. *Qualitative Research, 5*(4), 475–97.

Clegg, S., Tan, J. & Saeidi, S. (2002). Reflecting or acting? Reflective practice and continuing professional development in higher education. *Reflective Practice, 3*(1), 131–46.

Cohen, R. & Kennedy, P. T. (2007). *Global Sociology* (2nd edn). Basingstoke: Palgrave Macmillan.

de Craen, A. J. M., Roos, P. J., de Vries, A. L. & Kleijnen, J. (1996). Effect of colour of drugs: systematic review of perceived effect of drugs and their effectiveness. *British Medical Journal, 313*, 1624–6.

David, G. (2011). Interprofessional learning: reasons, judgement, and action. *Mind, Culture and Activity, 18*(4), 342.

DCSF (2009). *The Impact of the Commercial World on Children's Wellbeing.* Nottingham: Department for Culture, Schools and Families. Retrieved from https://www.education.gov.uk/publications/eOrderingDownload/00669-2009DOM-EN.pdf.

Dimond, B. (2008). *Legal Aspects of Nursing.* Harlow: Longman.

Dreyfus, H. L. & Dreyfus, S. E. (2009). The relationship of theory and practice in the acquisition of skill. In P. Benner, C. A. Chesla & C. A. Tanner (eds.), *Expertise in Nursing Practice: Caring, Clinical Judgement and Ethics* (2nd edn, pp. 1–24). New York: Springer Publishing Company.

Driscoll, J. (2000). *Practising Clinical Supervision.* London: Bailliere Tindall.

Edwards, G. & Thomas, G. (2010). Can reflective practice be taught? *Educational Studies, 36*(4), 403–14.

Felps, W., Mitchell, T. R. & Byington, E. (2006). How, when and why bad apples spoil the barrel: negative group members and dysfunctional groups. *Research in Organizational Behavior, 27*, 175–222.

Fleming, M. D. (2001). *Teaching and Learning Styles: VARK Strategies.* New Zealand: Honolulu Community College.

Fook, J. & Gardner, F. (2007). *Practising Critical Reflection: A Resource Handbook.* Maidenhead: Open University Press.

Gardner, K., Bridges, S. & Walmsley, D. (2012). International peer review in undergraduate dentistry: enhancing reflective practice in an online community of practice. *European Journal of Dental Education*, 16(4), 208–12.

Ghaye, T. & Lillyman, S. (2006). *Learning and Critical Incidents: Reflective Practice for Health Care Professionals* (2nd edn). Salisbury: Mark Allen Publishing.

Gibbs, G. (1988). *Learning by Doing: A Guide to Teaching and Learning Methods*. Oxford: Oxford Polytechnic, Further Education Unit.

Gilligan, C., Ward, J. V. McLean Taylor, J. & Bardige, B. (1988). *Mapping the Moral Domain: A Contribution of Woman's Thinking to Psychological Theory and Education*. Cambridge, MA: Harvard University Press.

Glaze, J. E. (2001). Reflection as a transforming process: student advanced nurse practitioners' experiences of developing reflective skills as part of an MSc programme. *Journal of Advanced Nursing*, 34(5), 639–47.

Glaze, J. E. (2002). Stages in coming to terms with reflection: student advanced nurse practitioners' perceptions of their reflective journeys. *Journal of Advanced Nursing*, 37(3), 265–72.

Glina, D. M. R., Cardoso, A. S., Isosaki, M. & Rocha, L. E. (2011). Participatory ergonomics: understanding the contributions of reflection groups in a hospital food service. *International Journal of Industrial Ergonomics*, 41, 96–105.

Graber, M. L. (2009). Educational strategies to reduce diagnostic error: can you teach this stuff? *Advances in Health Sciences Education: Theory and Practice*, 14(S1), 63–9.

Graham, M. & Schiele, J. H. (2010). Equality-of-oppressions and anti-discriminatory models in social work: reflections from the USA and UK. *European Journal of Social Work*, 13(2), 231–44.

Hakim, C. (2003). *Models of the Family in Modern Societies: Ideals and Realities*. Aldershot: Ashgate.

Hallam, J. (2000). *Nursing the Image: Media, Culture and Professional Identity*. London: Routledge.

Hargreaves, J. (2004). So how do you feel about that? Assessing reflective practice. *Nurse Education Today*, 24(3), 196–201.

Harold, P., Mark, M., Doug, R. & Robert, B. (2008). Learning styles: concepts and evidence. *Psychological Science in the Public Interest*, 9(3), 105.

Higgs, M. & Dulewicz, V. (2000). The seven elements of emotional intelligence. *Quality Focus*, 4(1), 4.

HMSO (2013). *Report of the Mid Staffordshire NHS Foundation Trust Public Inquiry*. London: The Stationery Office. Retrieved from www.midstaffspublicinquiry.com/report.

Hobbs, V. (2007). Faking it or hating it: can reflective practice be forced? *Reflective Practice*, 8(3), 405–17.

Honey, P. & Mumford, A. (1992). *The Manual of Learning Styles* (3rd edn). Maidenhead: Peter Honey.

Hook, D., Franks, B. & Bauer, M. W. (2011). *The Social Pyschology of Communication*. Basingstoke: Palgrave Macmillan.

Hudson Jones, A. (1988). *Images of Nursing*. Philadelphia: University of Pennsylvania Press.

Hursthouse, R. (1999). *On Virtue Ethics*. Oxford: Oxford University Press.

Iwama, M. (2006). *The Kawa Model: Culturally Relevant Occupational Therapy*. Philadelphia: Churchill Livingstone Elsevier.

Jenkins, G. W. & Tortora, G. J. (2013). *Anatomy & Physiology, from Science to Life* (3rd edn). Singapore: John Wiley & Sons.

Johns, C. (2009). *Becoming a Reflective Practitioner*. Chichester: Wiley-Blackwell.

Karban, K. & Smith, S. (2010). Developing critical reflection within an interprofessional learning programme. In H. Bradbury, N. Frost, S. Killminster & N. Zucas (eds.), *Beyond Reflective Practice* (pp. 170–81). Abingdon: Routledge.

Keyes, M. (2012). *The Mystery of Mercy Close*. London: Penguin Books.

Kiekkas, P. (2011). The role of non-blaming culture in learning from errors. *Nursing in Critical Care*, 16(1), 3–4.

King, S. (2001). *On Writing*. London: Hodder & Stoughton.

Koonce, T. Y., Giuse, N. B. & Storrow, A. B. (2011). A pilot study to evaluate learning style-tailored information prescriptions for hypertensive emergency department patients. *Journal of the Medical Library Association: JMLA*, 99(4), 280.

Lai, G. & Calandra, B. (2010). Examining the effects of computer-based scaffolds on novice teachers' reflective journal writing. *Educational Technology Research and Development*, 58(4), 421–37.

Le Fanu, J. (1999). *The Rise and Fall of Modern Medicine*. London: Little, Brown and Company.

Lepine, J. A. & Van-Dyne, L. (2001). Peer responses to low performers: an attributional model of helping in the context of groups. *Academy of Management Review*, 26(1), 67–84.

Lewis, D. B. (2001). *Whistle Blowing at Work*. London: The Athlone Press.

Lindstrom, M. (2011). *Brandwashed: The Tricks Companies Use to Manipulate Our Minds and Persuade Us to Buy*. New York: Crown Business.

Litchfield, A., Frawley, J. & Nettleton, S. (2010). Contextualising and integrating into the curriculum the learning and teaching of work-ready professional graduate attributes. *Higher Education Research and Development*, 29(5), 519–34.

Macfarlane, B. & Gourlay, L. (2009). The reflection game: enacting the penitent self. *Teaching in Higher Education*, 14(4), 455–9.

Macionis, J. J. (2010). *Sociology*. Boston: Pearson Education.

MacLeod, M. L. P. (1996). *Practising Nursing: Becoming Experienced*. Edinburgh: Churchill Livingstone.

Mamede, S., Schmidt, H. G. & Penaforte, J. C. (2008). Effects of reflective practice on the accuracy of medical diagnoses. *Medical Education*, 42(5), 468–75.

Mamede, S., Schmidt, H. G. & Rikers, R. (2007). Diagnostic errors and reflective practice in medicine. *Journal of Evaluation in Clinical Practice*, 13(1), 138–45.

Mann, K., Gordon, J. & MacLeod, A. (2009). Reflection and reflective practice in health professions education: a systematic review. *Advances in Health Science Education*, 14, 595–621.

Mantell, A. & Scragg, T. (2011). *Safeguarding Adults in Social Work* (2nd edn). Exeter: Learning Matters.

Mantzoukas, S. & Watkinson, S. (2008). Redescribing reflective practice and evidence-based practice discourses. *International Journal of Nursing Practice*, 14(2), 129–34.

McCracken, S. G. & Marsh, J. C. (2008). Practitioner expertise in evidence-based practice decision making. *Research on Social Work Practice*, 18(4), 301–10.

McMillan, K. & Weyers, J. (2006). *The Smarter Student, Skills and Strategies for Success at University*. Harlow: Pearson Education Limited.

Mezirow, J. (1990). *Fostering Critical Reflection in Adulthood: A Guide to Transformative and Emancipatory Learning*. San Francisco: Jossey-Bass.

Miceli, M. P. & Near, J. P. (2002). What makes whistle blowers effective? Three field studies. *Human Relations*, 55, 455–79.

Miller, S. (2005). What it's like being the 'holder of the space': a narrative on working with reflective practice in groups. *Reflective Practice*, 6(3), 367–77.

Montgomery, L. A. (2003). Digital portfolios in teacher education: blending professional standards, assessment, technology, and reflective practice. *Computers in the Schools*, 20(1–2), 171–86.

Moon, J. A. (2006). *Learning Journals: A Handbook for Reflective Practice and Professional Development*. Abingdon: Routledge.

O'Hagan, K. (2007). *Competence in Social Work Practice: A Practical*

Guide for Students and Professionals. London: Jessica Kingsley Publishers.

Packard, V. (2007). *The Hidden Persuaders.* Brooklyn: Mark Crispin Miller.

Pau, A. K. H. & Croucher, R. (2003). The use of PBL to facilitate the development of professional attributes in second year dental students. *European Journal of Dental Education, 7*(3), 123–9.

Pirie, M. (2009). *101 Great Philosophers.* London: Continuum.

Platzer, H., Blake, D. & Ashford, D. (2000). Barriers to learning from reflection: a study of the use of groupwork with post-registration nurses. *Journal of Advanced Nursing, 31*(5), 1001–8.

Plummer, K. (2001). *Documents of Life 2* (2nd edn). London: Sage.

Purlito, R. (2011). *Ethical Dimensions in the Health Professions* (5th edn). Missouri: Elsevier Saunders Company.

Rhine, S. & Bryant, J. (2007). Enhancing pre-service teachers' reflective practice with digital video-based dialogue. *Reflective Practice, 8*(3), 345–58.

Rodham, K. (2010). *Health Psychology.* Basingstoke: Palgrave Macmillan.

Rogers, W. & Ballantyne, A. (2010). Towards a practical definition of professional behaviour. *Journal of Medical Ethics, 36,* 250–4.

Rolfe, G., Jasper, M. & Freshwater, D. (2011). *Critical Reflection in Practice: Generating Knowledge for Care* (2nd edn). Basingstoke: Palgrave Macmillan.

Ross, J. (2011). Traces of self: online reflective practices and performances in higher education. *Teaching in Higher Education, 16*(1), 113–26.

Russell, T. (2005). Can reflective practice be taught? *Reflective Practice, 6*(2), 199–204.

Sandars, J. & Murray, C. (2011). Digital storytelling to facilitate reflective learning in medical students. *Medical Education, 45*(6), 649.

Sanderson, H. (2011). Using learning styles in information literacy: critical considerations for librarians. *The Journal of Academic Librarianship, 37*(5), 376–85.

Schön, D. A. (1991). *The Reflective Practitioner: How Professionals Think in Action.* Aldershot: Arena, Ashgate Publishing.

Skivenes, M. & Trygstad, S. C. (2010). When whistle-blowing works: the Norwegian case. *Human Relations, 63*(7), 1071–97.

Smith, E. (2011). Teaching critical reflection. *Teaching in Higher Education, 16*(2), 211–23.

Somers, M. & Casal, J. C. (2011). Type of wrongdoing and whistle-blowing: further evidence that type of wrongdoing affects the whistle-blowing process. *Public Personnel Management*, 40(2), 151–64.

Stewart, J. (2012). Reflecting on reflection: increasing health and social care students' engagement and enthusiasm for reflection. *Reflective Practice: International and Multidisciplinary Perspectives*, 13(5), 719–33.

Swann, W. B. J., Johnson, R. E. & Bosson, J. K. (2009). Identity negotiation at work. *Research in Organizational Behavior*, 29, 81–109.

Thomas, P. A. & Goldberg, H. (2007). Tracking reflective practice-based learning by medical students during an ambulatory clerkship. *Journal of General Internal Medicine*, 22(11), 1583–6.

Thompson, N. (2009). *People Skills* (3rd edn). Basingstoke: Palgrave Macmillan.

Thompson, N. & Pascal, J. (2012). Developing critically reflective practice. *Reflective Practice: International and Multidisciplinary Perspectives*, 13(2), 311–25.

Thornton, T. (2008). Values based practice and reflective judgement. *Philosophy, Psychiatry, & Psychology*, 15(2), 125–33.

Tileston, D. W. (2005). *10 Best Teaching Practices* (2nd edn). Thousand Oaks, CA: Sage.

Trongmateerut, P. & Sweeney, J. T. (2012). The influence of subjective norms on whistle-blowing: a cross-cultural investigation. *Journal of Business Ethics*, 112(3), 437–51.

van Mook, W. N. K. A., van Luijk, S. J., O'Sullivan, H., Wass, V., Schuwirth, L. W. & van der Vleuten, C. P. M. (2009). General considerations regarding assessment of professional behaviour. *European Journal of Internal Medicine*, 20(4), e90–e95.

Wald, H. S. & Reis, S. P. (2010). Beyond the margins: reflective writing and development of reflective capacity in medical education. *Journal of General Internal Medicine*, 25(7), 746–9.

Wharton, S. (2012). Presenting a united front: assessed reflective writing on a group experience. *Reflective Practice: International and Multidisciplinary Perspectives*, 13(4), 489–501.

WHO (2010). *Framework for Action on Interprofessional Education & Collaborative Practice*. Geneva: WHO. Retrieved from http://whqlib doc.who.int/hq/2010/WHO_HRH_HPN_10.3_eng.pdf.

Index

Milton Keynes UK
Ingram Content Group UK Ltd.
UKHW020650130824
446857UK00011B/179